The Battle Against Malaria: A Historical and Scientific Exploration

Lemony

First Printing, 2024

CONTENTS

CHAPTER I: INTRODUCTION AND LITERATURE REVIEW

1.1. An introduction to malaria 2

1.2. A brief history of malaria 2

1.3. Malaria today and current treatment 3

1.4. A summary of the *Plasmodium falciparum* lifecycle 5

1.5. Haemozoin formation and inhibition 6

1.6. Chloroquine and chloroquine resistance 9

1.7. Reversed chloroquines 11

  1.7.1. Dibemequines 12

1.7.2. Pyridodibemequines and their metabolites 13

1.10. Introduction to research project and rationale 19

1.11. Aims 21

1.12. Objectives 21

CHAPTER II: BIOANALYTICAL METHOD DEVELOPMENT AND VALIDATION

2.1. INTRODUCTION 23

  2.1.1. Chapter aims 23

  2.1.2. Bioanalytical techniques 23

    2.1.2.1. Reversed-phase high-performance liquid chromatography 23

2.1.2.2. Mass spectrometry 25

2.1.2.3. Sample preparation 27

2.1.3. Method validation 28

2.1.3.1. Calibration curve 28

2.1.3.2. Internal standard 30

2.1.3.3. Accuracy 30

2.1.3.4. Precision 30

2.1.3.5. Selectivity 30

2.1.3.6. Sensitivity 31

2.1.3.7. Acceptance criteria for an analytical batch 31

2.1.3.8. Carryover 31

2.1.3.9. Matrix effects 32

2.1.3.10. Analyte stability 33

2.2.4. Pyridodibemequine parent and metabolite analytical chemistry 33

2.2. METHODS 37

2.2.1. Materials 37

2.2.2. Instrumentation 38

2.2.3. Bioanalytical method development 39

2.2.3.1. Mass spectrometry 39

2.2.3.2. Reversed-phase chromatography 39

2.2.3.3. Sample preparation 39

2.2.4. Bioanalytical method validation 40

2.2.4.1. Calibration curve 41

2.2.4.2. Selectivity 45

2.2.4.3. Sensitivity 46

2.2.4.4. Carryover 46

2.2.4.5. Matrix effects 46

2.2.4.6. Stock solution stability 47

2.2.4.7. Working solution stability 48

2.2.4.8. Bench-top biological matrix stability 49

2.2.4.9. Post-preparative stability 49

2.2.4.10. Dosing vehicle stability 50

2.3. RESULTS AND DISCUSSION 51

2.3.1. Bioanalytical method development and partial validation for the pharmacokinetic studies in healthy mice 51

2.3.1.1. Mass spectrometry 51

2.3.1.2. Chromatography 54

2.3.1.3. Sample preparation 56

2.3.1.4. Selectivity 57

2.3.1.5. Sensitivity 58

2.3.1.6. Carryover 60

2.3.1.7. Calibration curve 62

2.3.1.8. Matrix effects 64

2.3.1.9. Stock solution stability 66

2.3.1.10. Working solution stability 67

2.3.1.11. Bench-top biological matrix stability 68

2.3.1.12. Post-preparative stability 70

2.3.1.13. Oral formulation stability 71

2.3.1.14. Intravenous formulation stability 72

2.3.2. Bioanalytical method development and partial validation for the pharmacokinetic studies in malaria-infected mice 73

2.3.2.1. Mass spectrometry 74

2.3.2.2. Chromatography 75

2.3.2.3. Sample preparation 78

2.3.2.4. Selectivity 79

2.3.2.5. Sensitivity 80

2.3.2.6. Carryover 81

2.3.2.7. Calibration curve 82

2.3.2.8. Matrix effects 84

2.3.2.9. Bench-top biological matrix stability 85

2.3.2.10. Post-preparative stability 86

2.4. CONCLUSION 87

CHAPTER III: IN VIVO PHARMACOKINETICS IN A HEALTHY MURINE MODEL

3.1. INTRODUCTION 89

3.1.1. Chapter aim 89

3.1.2. Absorption, distribution, metabolism, and excretion 89

3.1.3. Absorption, distribution, metabolism, and excretion of the parent pyridodibemequines and major metabolites 92

3.1.4. A review of non-compartmental analysis 95

3.1.5. Determinants for compound progression 98

3.1.6. Pharmacokinetic study design in healthy mice 98

3.2. METHODS 101

3.2.1. Ethics statement 101

3.2.2. Animal housing 101

3.2.3. Materials and instrumentation 101

3.2.4. Compound administration and sampling 101

3.2.5. Analyte quantification 102

3.2.6. Non-compartmental pharmacokinetic analysis 103

3.3. RESULTS AND DISCUSSION 105

3.3.1. Review of the bioanalytical method performance 105

3.3.2. Pharmacokinetics of the *ortho*-substituted parent compound **49** 106

3.3.3. Pharmacokinetics of the *ortho*-substituted metabolite **49M1** 110

3.3.4. Pharmacokinetics of the *ortho*-substituted metabolite **49M2** 112

3.3.5. Pharmacokinetics of the *meta*-substituted parent **43** 115

3.3.6. Pharmacokinetics of the *meta*-substituted metabolite **43M1** 118

3.3.7. Pharmacokinetics of the *meta*-substituted metabolite **43M2** 121

3.3.8. Pharmacokinetics of the *para*-substituted parent compound **47** 123

3.3.9. Pharmacokinetics of the *para*-substituted metabolite **47M1** 126

3.3.10. *In vitro-in vivo* absorption, distribution, metabolism, and elimination relationship 129

3.3.11. Lead candidate selection 129

3.4. CONCLUSION 131

CHAPTER IV: IN VIVO PHARMACOKINETICS AND PHARMACODYNAMICS IN A MALARIA-INFECTED MURINE MODEL

4.1. INTRODUCTION 133

4.1.1. Chapter aim 133

4.1.2. A brief introduction to pharmacodynamics 133

4.1.3. The *Plasmodium falciparum*-infected humanised murine model 134

4.1.4. Pharmacokinetic and pharmacodynamic study design in a malaria-infected murine model 138

4.2. METHODS 140

4.2.1. Ethics statement 140

4.2.2. Animal housing 140

4.2.3. Materials and instrumentation 140

4.2.4. Engraftment and infection in humanised mice 141

4.2.5. Compound administration and sampling 143

4.2.6. Pharmacodynamic analysis 143

4.2.7. Pharmacokinetic analysis 144

4.3. RESULTS AND DISCUSSION 146

4.3.1. Review of the *in vivo* efficacy experimental procedure 146

4.3.2. Review of the bioanalytical method performance 146

4.3.3. Pharmacokinetics and pharmacodynamics of **43M1** 147

4.3.4. Pharmacokinetics and pharmacodynamics of **47M1** 151

4.3.5. Review of the pharmacokinetics and pharmacodynamics of the lead pyridodibemequine candidates 155

4.4. CONCLUSION 160

CHAPTER V: IN VITRO COMBINATIONS WITH CLINICALLY RELEVANT ANTIMALARIALS

5.1. INTRODUCTION 162

5.1.1. Chapter aim 162

5.1.2. Combination therapy 162

5.1.3. A short mechanistic review of selected antimalarial agents 164

5.1.3.1. Chloroquine 164

5.1.3.2. Dihydroartemisinin 165

5.1.3.3. Mefloquine 166

5.1.3.4. Lumefantrine 167

5.1.3.5. Methylene blue 167

5.1.3.6. Atovaquone 168

5.1.4. Fixed-dose ratio isobolograms 168

5.1.5. *In vitro* antimalarial isobologram study design 170

5.2. METHODS 172

5.2.1. *In vitro* continuous culture of *Plasmodium falciparum* 172

5.2.2. *In vitro* antiplasmodial assays 172

5.2.2.1. Single compound antiplasmodial assay 173

5.2.2.2. Fixed-ratio isobologram assay 174

5.3. RESULTS AND DISCUSSION 177

5.3.1. Single compound antiplasmodial activity 177

5.3.2. Combinations with chloroquine 177

5.3.3. Combinations with dihydroartemisinin 180

5.3.4. Combinations with mefloquine 184

5.3.5. Combinations with lumefantrine 188

5.3.6. Combinations with methylene blue 191

5.3.7. Combinations with atovaquone 194

5.3.8. Study limitations 197

5.4. CONCLUSION 198

CHAPTER VI: CONCLUSIONS AND FUTURE STUDIES

6. CONCLUSIONS AND FUTURE STUDIES 200

6.1. Conclusions 200

6.2. Future studies 204

CHAPTER VII: REFERENCES 207

CHAPTER I

INTRODUCTION AND LITERATURE REVIEW

1.1. An introduction to malaria

Malaria is an infectious disease caused by the protozoan *Plasmodium.* These parasites are transmitted by an infected female *Anopheles* mosquito which can transfer five species of *Plasmodium* to humans namely; *P. vivax*, *P. ovale*, *P. malariae*, *P. knowlesi* and, the most threatening, *P. falciparum* which culminates in the highest human mortality. During the course of its lifecycle within the human, *Plasmodium* continually infects and ruptures the host erythrocyte which manifests in the clinical symptoms and complications of malaria such as fever, chills, cerebral malaria, and anaemia and if left untreated will result in fatality[1,2].

1.2. A brief history of malaria

Direct evidence of malaria in humans dates as far back as 3200 BC, as demonstrated by a malaria parasite antigen that was detected in preserved Egyptian mummies[3]. Ancient records and artefacts dating from 2700 BC and onwards have referenced the now established symptomatic stages of malaria[4]. The term malaria derives from the Italian "mal'aria" which translates to "bad air" and refers to the historical idea that the air surrounding stagnant water had malignancies which caused the symptoms of malaria. Although the history of malaria extends far back in time, the scientific understanding of malaria only began to grow at the end of the late 19th century[4,5]. In 1880, Charles L. A. Laveran discovered the intraerythrocytic parasite, *Plasmodium*, as the causal agent for malaria[6]. In 1897, Ronald Ross demonstrated that malaria was transmitted by mosquitos and in 1900, Patrick Mason provided further evidence that the *Anopheles* mosquito is the vector for transmission[7,8].

Natural products were used as the earliest therapeutic intervention against malaria. The first effective treatment for malaria was introduced around 1640. This was an extract prepared from the bark of the *Cinchona* tree which contained the active ingredient quinine belonging to the quinoline group of compounds[9]. In the 1940s, a synthetic quinoline alternative named chloroquine (CQ) started to replace quinine as the primary treatment for malaria. CQ was widely used due to its efficacy, safety, and low cost until the extensive emergence of CQ resistance which rendered the drug ineffective[10]. From 1945, proguanil and other antifolate derivatives, such as pyrimethamine, were discovered; however, their use as monotherapy resulted in the rapid propagation of resistant strains[11,12]. In the 1970s, artemisinin (ART), derived from the *Artemsia annua* plant, started to replace CQ as the first-line antimalarial treatment[13]. **Figure 1.1** displays the chemical structures of the antimalarials introduced above.

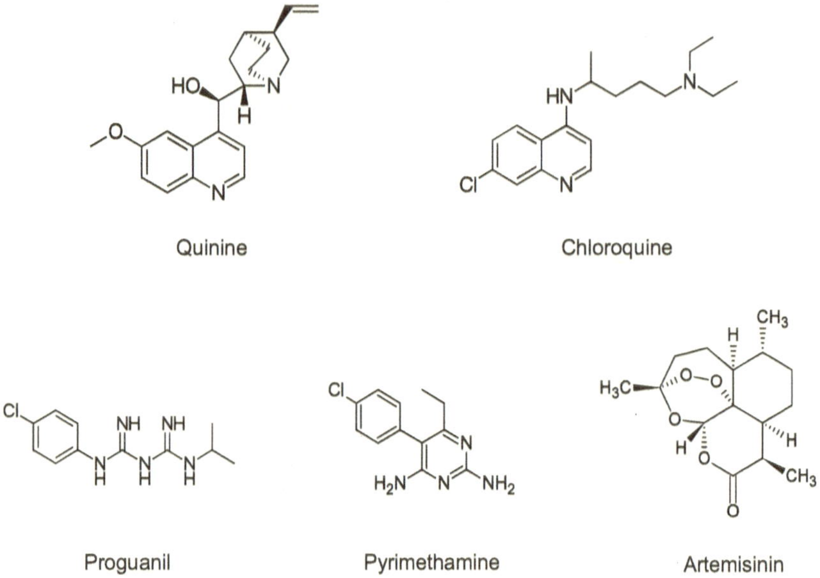

Quinine Chloroquine

Proguanil Pyrimethamine Artemisinin

Figure 1.1. Chemical structures of quinine and CQ belonging to the quinoline class of compounds, proguanil and pyrimethamine belonging to the antifolate group, and ART.

1.3. Malaria today and current treatment

The World Health Organisation (WHO) reported 228 million cases of malaria globally in 2018, with the largest burden occurring in Africa, followed by Southeast Asia. Pregnant women and children are the most vulnerable to this disease which claimed an estimated 405000 lives in 2018[1]. **Figure 1.2** presents the geographic distribution of the incidence of malaria in 2018. Malaria also has a high economic impact as a result of the cost of healthcare, decreased productivity, and the loss of investment, amongst other factors. In 2018, 2.7 billion US dollars was globally invested in malaria control and elimination efforts[1,14]. It is crucial to develop effective treatments to ultimately alleviate morbidity and mortality as well as relieve the economic pressure caused by this disease.

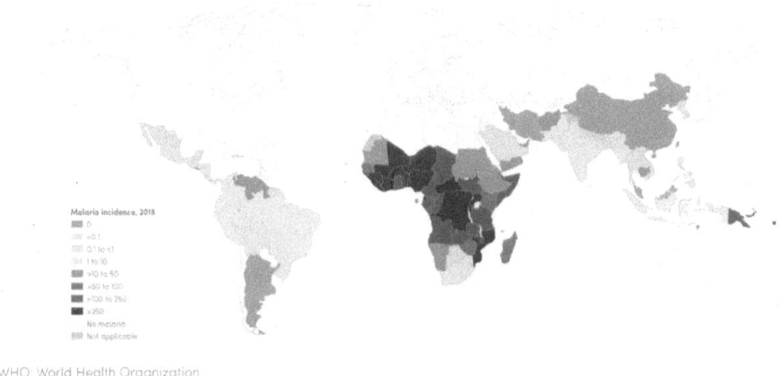

Figure 1.2. Malaria case incidence rate depicting the number of cases per 1000 population at risk in 2018. Figure reproduced from the World Malaria Report 2019 with permission from WHO under the Creative Commons Attribution License[1].

Preventative intervention against malaria includes vector control through insecticide-treated mosquito nets and antimalarial prophylaxis. For the treatment of malaria, the use of antimalarials as a single entity is not recommended due to the increased risk of drug resistance. The incorporation of two or more drugs, each with distinct molecular targets, is often administered to delay the onset of resistance and reduce treatment failure. The WHO recommends ART-based combination therapy as the first-line treatment for uncomplicated malaria. This regimen pairs a fast-acting, rapidly eliminated ART derivative, such as artesunate, artemether, or dihydroartemisinin (DHA), with a longer-acting, slowly eliminated partner drug which can diminish persisting parasites, such as piperaquine, mefloquine (MEF), or lumefantrine (LUM)[1,15,16]. A summarised mechanistic evaluation of selected clinically relevant antimalarials is presented in **Chapter V, Section 5.1.3**.

Concerted efforts towards malaria eradication have resulted in an approximate 30% decrease in the global number of deaths and an 11 million reduction in the number of cases from 2010–2018[1]. Despite these progressions, investment towards disease management should not be alleviated as there still exists the risk of resistance emerging towards the current frontline therapy, which could result in a significant hinderance to disease control. ART resistance has already been observed in Southeast Asia where parasites have displayed delayed clearance to ART-based therapies[17,18]. Consequently, there has been a resurgence in antimalarial drug discovery programmes which has led to the identification of several new therapeutic agents which are at various stages of preclinical and clinical development[19,20]. Additionally, significant progress has been made towards RTS,S/AS01, the first licensed vaccine against *P. falciparum*. A phase 3 clinical trial demonstrated partial efficacy of RTS,S/AS01 in young infants and children and a pilot study is currently underway in Ghana, Kenya, and Malawi to further evaluate the vaccine for wider implementation. However, given the limited protective immunity of the vaccine against *P. falciparum*, vector control and chemotherapy measures are still required[1,21].

To this end, the research presented in this study focuses on the preclinical evaluation of a novel series of antimalarial compounds.

1.4. A summary of the *Plasmodium falciparum* lifecycle

The *P. falciparum* lifecycle has two distinct parts, the sexual lifecycle within the female *Anopheles* mosquito vector and the asexual and sexual lifecycles within the human host[22]. **Figure 1.3** depicts a summary of the *P. falciparum* lifecycle. Fertilised *P. falciparum* gametocytes develop from oocytes into infectious haploid sporozoites outside the gut wall of the mosquito. Upon maturity, the sporozoites channel to the mosquito's salivary glands and the contaminated saliva is transferred to a human during the course of the mosquito's blood meal. The transmitted sporozoites travel through the human's circulatory system and are transported to the liver where they invade the hepatocytes. The sporozoites remain within the hepatocytes for five to ten days. During this period, they mature into schizonts and further develop to produce tens of thousands of haploid merozoites, which elicits the rupture of the schizont resulting in the release of the merozoites into systemic circulation. The asexual blood-stage of the lifecycle begins when the merozoite infects an erythrocyte. The intraerythrocytic merozoite enlarges and differentiates to produce an immature trophozoite which is referred to as a ring-stage parasite, as its morphology resembles that of a circular band. The ring-phase parasite undergoes active metabolism and develops into a mature trophozoite. This stage is referred to as the trophozoite stage and is predominately associated with haemoglobin ingestion and degradation. Then, the trophozoite undergoes maturation and nuclear division and develops into a schizont. Differentiation of the schizont produces merozoites which burst out of the erythrocyte. The merozoites then proceed to invade uninfected erythrocytes, and the blood-stage cycle continues[23,24,25,26].

The sexual stage of the lifecycle occurs when a small percentage of the ring-phase parasites develop into infectious gametocytes. During its blood meal, the female *Anopheles* mosquito may ingest the gametocyte-infected erythrocytes. The parasites are then transferred to the mosquito where sexual maturation can commence and subsequently, successive cycles of human infection can occur[23,24,25,27].

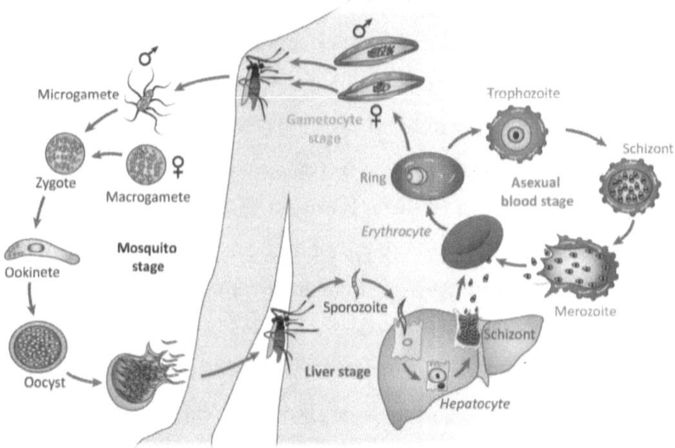

Figure 1.3. *P. falciparum* lifecycles within the female *Anopheles* mosquito and the human host. Figure reproduced from Maier, A., Matuschewski, K., Zhang, M. & Rug, M. *Plasmodium falciparum. Trends in Parasitology* **35**, 481-482 (2019). Copyright (2019) Elsevier.

1.5. Haemozoin formation and inhibition

P. falciparum ingests and degrades haemoglobin amassed within the erythrocyte. Haemoglobin accounts for approximately 95% of the proteins found within the erythrocytic cytoplasm and up to 75% of this is consumed by the parasite[23,28]. Trophozoite-stage parasites are primarily responsible for haemoglobin metabolism as compared to ring- and schizont-stage parasites[29,30]. Parasitic haemoglobin digestion occurs through a cytostomal system which spans the membrane that separates the parasitic cytoplasm from the erythrocytic cytoplasm. Cytostomes engulf erythrocytic haemoglobin-enriched cytoplasm and form vesicles within the parasite through cytostomal budding. These vesicles appear to coalesce, resulting in the formation of a digestive vacuole (DV). The recurrent vesicle production and fusion of the vesicle and DV membranes enable continuous delivery of haemoglobin into the DV[31,32].

The DV is a single-membrane enclosed organelle and is the major site for haemoglobin catabolism. The intra-organelle pH of the DV is maintained in an acidic state between 5.0 and 5.4[33,34]. Haemoglobin proteolysis releases globin and haem. Globin is further hydrolysed to produce amino acids which are incorporated into proteins synthesised by the parasite. The ferrous iron centre of the released haem autooxidises in the acidic DV which subsequently produces ferriprotoporphyrin IX (FPIX); this ferric state of iron is achieved through the liberation of electrons which are believed to react with oxygen to produce reactive oxygen species. The parasite resolves this oxidative stress through dismutase and catalase reactions[23,35]. The FPIX that is generated presents a potentially toxic effect on the parasite since it is capable of permeabilising membranes which consequently promotes cell lysis[36,37,38]. Under normal physiological conditions, the parasite is able to attenuate the reactive FPIX through dimerisation followed by crystallisation of FPIX dimers, producing an inert biocrystal called haemozoin[39,40,41,42]. Haemozoin or its synthetic form β-haematin, originally called malarial pigment, is a distinctive characteristic of malaria-infected erythrocytes. An in-depth analysis of haemozoin has shown that the crystal is composed entirely of FPIX. Additionally, it has been demonstrated that the majority of toxic FPIX that is produced during haemoglobin degradation is sequestered as haemozoin[41,43]. **Figure 1.4** displays a summary of haemoglobin metabolism inside a *P. falciparum*-infected erythrocyte.

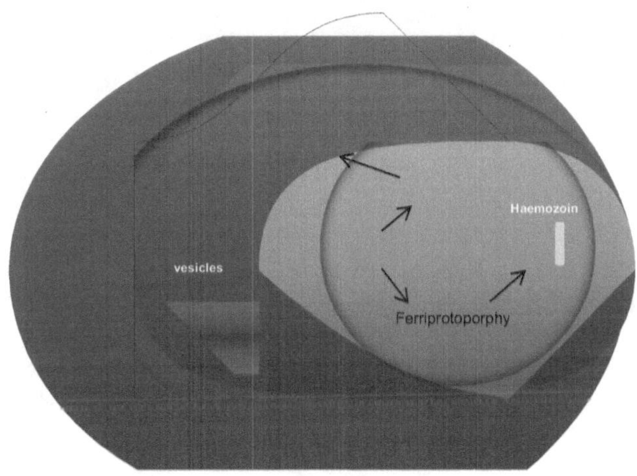

Figure 1.4. Summary of haemoglobin degradation and haemozoin formation with intraerythrocytic *P. falciparum.*

Cognisant of the critical role of haemozoin synthesis in allowing parasite survival, targeting and preventing this essential detoxification process provides an appealing opportunity to combat the parasite. In this regard, various antimalarials have been shown to inhibit the formation of haemozoin, leading to the accumulation of destructive levels of FPIX, which kills the parasite. The mechanism of preventing FPIX detoxification is proposed to result from interference by haemozoin-inhibiting drugs with both FPIX and haemozoin. It has been shown these drugs can bind to FPIX, creating a complex which consequently is hypothesised to prevent further FPIX crystallisation[44,45,46,47]. Additionally, it has been demonstrated that the FPIX-drug complex or free drug can adsorb onto the face of haemozoin which is subsequently postulated to hinder further crystal growth[40,42,48]. The formation of the FPIX-drug and haemozoin-drug complexes ultimately results in a toxic accumulation of FPIX and drug-bound FPIX[49].

In order to definitively characterise a drug as a haemozoin inhibitor, a cellular haem fractionation assay was developed which measures the levels of FPIX and haemozoin present in trophozoites that have been incubated with increasing concentrations of a drug or experimental compound. Drugs which behave as haemozoin inhibitors display a significant dose-dependent increase in FPIX, which correlates to a decrease in haemozoin and corresponds to decreased parasite survival compared to the negative control[50]. This assay has been extended from CQ to other relevant antimalarials to elucidate whether haemozoin inhibition is their predominant mechanism of action. It was shown that CQ causes a concentration-dependent increase in FPIX, which correlates to parasite death and, therefore, provides direct evidence that CQ is a haemozoin inhibitor[51].

1.6. Chloroquine and chloroquine resistance

CQ is a 4-amino-7-chloroquinoline antimalarial drug which belongs to the quinoline family of compounds. Quinolines are heterocyclic compounds composed of a fused benzene and pyridine ring. CQ was widely used from the mid-1940s to the 1990s until the widespread emergence of chloroquine-resistant (CQR) strains, which led to the loss of its clinical efficacy[52].

CQ inhibits the FPIX crystallisation pathway within the DV and acts on the trophozoite stage of the parasite lifecycle when host haemoglobin digestion is at its peak[51]. CQ is a weak base which enters the parasite in its neutral form and passively diffuses down the pH gradient into the DV. CQ protonates at the quinoline nitrogen and at the tertiary amino group on the side chain upon entry into the acidic DV. In its charged form, CQ is less membrane permeable and is, therefore, unable to diffuse out of the DV, consequently, concentrating CQ at its site of action[53,54]. This is significant because it has been demonstrated that the accumulation of CQ within the DV is essential for its activity[55]. In addition to pH trapping, the high-affinity binding of CQ to FPIX is also postulated to contribute to the accumulation of CQ within the DV although, in this bound form, CQ is unlikely to exert its antiplasmodial activity[56,57].

An investigation into the structure-activity relationship (SAR) of CQ, as displayed in **Figure 1.5**, demonstrated that the 4-aminoquinoline core is necessary for FPIX binding and the 7-chloro group on the quinoline ring is a requirement for inhibiting β-haematin formation. Furthermore, the terminal nitrogen on the side chain and the quinoline nitrogen were identified to assist in DV accumulation by pH trapping[55]. In summary, the SAR studies suggest that CQ antiplasmodial activity is dependent on the degree of β-haematin inhibition due to the strength of complex formation with FPIX, as well as the magnitude of drug accumulation within the DV due to pH trapping[55,58].

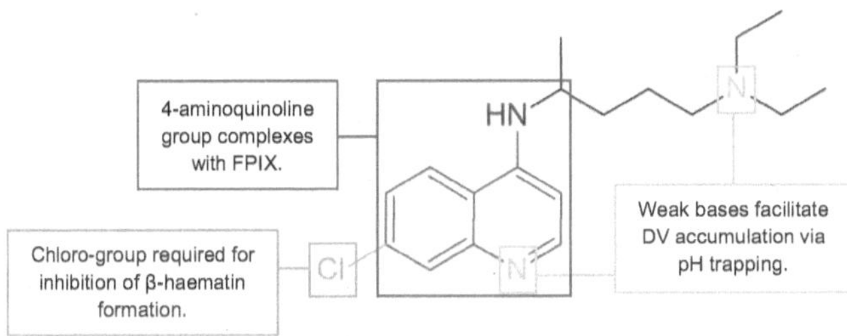

Figure 1.5. Proposed SAR of the 4-amino-7-chloroquinoline haemozoin inhibitor CQ[55].

CQ resistance is associated with polymorphisms in the *P. falciparum* chloroquine resistance transporter (PfCRT) protein which is a member of the drug/metabolite transporter superfamily. The gene *pfcrt* encodes a 424 amino acid protein which traverses the DV membrane[59,60]. Mutations in *pfcrt* are responsible for CQ resistance; of particular importance is the substitution mutation of lysine with threonine at position 76 (K76T) which is consistently present in almost all CQR strains and is, therefore, regarded as the primary determinant for CQ resistance[61]. K76T is located towards the vacuolar side of PfCRT and results in the loss of a positive charge from the presumed CQ substrate-binding site on PfCRT. In chloroquine-sensitive (CQS) strains, protonated CQ is unable to interact with the positively charged substrate-binding site on PfCRT which prevents its movement out of the DV. However, in CQR strains, the substrate-binding site is altered by the loss of a positive charge, due to the substitution of lysine with threonine, which allows protonated CQ to interact and bind with PfCRT and, subsequently, be transported down its electrochemical gradient. The efflux of CQ away from its site of action allows the parasite to control the FPIX detoxification process as it is no longer hindered by CQ accumulation[59,60,62].

CQ egress by CQR PfCRT was directly demonstrated using the *Xenopus laevis* oocyte expression system. This model expresses PfCRT at the plasma membrane of *X. laevis* oocytes and allows the movement of drugs to be studied by directly measuring the transfer of the drug from the mildly-acidic extracellular medium into the oocyte cytosol, which correlates to the efflux of drug from the parasite's DV to the cytosol. It was shown that CQR PfCRT transported protonated CQ into the oocyte cytosol whereas CQS PfCRT was unable to dissipate protonated CQ from the acidic compartment[63]. Additionally, it was shown that CQR parasites accumulate relatively less CQ in the DV compared to CQS parasites[64]. Together these findings underlie the differences in the CQ efflux mechanisms of CQS and CQR forms of PfCRT and further, it suggests that the mechanism of CQ resistance is not a result of changes in the drug target but rather a ramification of the variability of drug accumulation within the DV. Compensatory mutations in other transporter proteins, such as *P. falciparum* multidrug resistance (PfMDR)1, have also been associated with CQ resistance, but only in strains harbouring the CQR PfCRT genetic background. PfMDR1 is not directly responsible for CQR although it does alter a resistant parasite's susceptibility towards CQ[65].

1.7. Reversed chloroquines

Drug resistance is a major threat to malaria eradication and as evidence for ART resistance emerges, there is a need for novel therapeutic approaches which address this issue. One such strategy that has been explored is CQ-resistance reversal agents which are able to chemosensitise CQR strains of *P. falciparum*. A range of structurally-diverse drugs, whose clinical application excludes that of malaria, have been shown to restore the susceptibility of CQ in CQR strains of *P. falciparum*[17,66].

Verapamil and imipramine, amongst many others, have been identified as CQ-resistance reversers as they are able to inhibit PfCRT-mediated CQ extrusion from the DV, thereby circumventing the parasite's resistance mechanism. Although these drugs appeared promising, they were not further developed for this intended application as they require unsuitably high concentrations to exert their CQ-resistance reversing effect. To address this issue, it was proposed that the resistance reversing agent can be linked to a CQ-like molecule[67,68,69].

Since CQ accumulates within the DV, due to weak base pH trapping and FPIX binding, if the reversal agent is appended to the quinoline core, it could possibly enhance the accumulation of the reversal agent within the DV as well as deliver the reversal agent and the pharmacophore in a 1:1 ratio. Another suggested advantage of coupling two separately active moieties into one molecule is that the oral absorption of the two entities would match to allow simultaneous systemic delivery. The feasibility of these hybrid compounds or reversed CQs was explored, and they were shown to be effective against CQR parasites[70,71]. Thus, this novel class of reversed CQs was developed. These dual functioning compounds integrate antimalarial activity with CQ-resistance reversing mechanisms and are intended for combination therapy in adjunct with CQ against CQR strains of *P. falciparum*[71]. The CQ-like core is responsible for eliciting antimalarial activity and the resistance reversing group has been shown to interact and bind to PfCRT in a manner which inhibits the egress of CQ from the DV, thereby negating the parasite's CQ-resistance mechanism and subsequently potentiating the activity of CQ against the CQR strain. Evidence suggests competitive binding between CQ and the reversing group for the proposed CQ binding site on PfCRT[72].

1.7.1. Dibemequines

Dibemequines (DBQs) are a series of reversed CQ derivatives that inhibit haemozoin formation and chemosensitise CQR strains by obstructing CQ transport by the CQR PfCRT. These compounds incorporate the proposed pharmacophores of a reversed CQ, namely a 4-amino-7-chloroquinoline core which is linked via a methylene bridge to a resistance reversing dibenzylmethylamine side chain. **Figure 1.6** illustrates compound **36**, an analogue from the DBQ series, which was shown to be equally active in both CQS and CQR strains of *P. falciparum*. The increased susceptibility of **36** in the CQR strain compared to that of CQ suggests that there is an absence of cross-resistance between **36** and CQ[73,74].

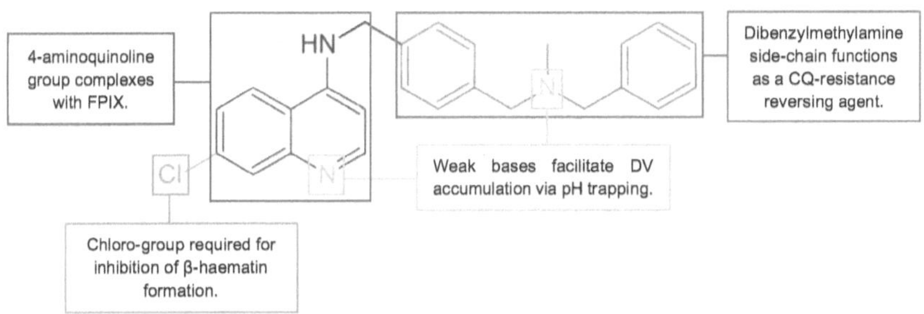

Figure 1.6. Proposed SAR of the resistance reversing DBQ **36**[55,73].

Compound **36** was shown to inhibit haemozoin formation, and the proposed SAR of CQ suggests that the 4-amino-7-chloroquinoline core of **36** is responsible for its observed antiplasmodial activity[75]. *In vitro* isobologram analyses were performed to evaluate the CQ chemosensitising potential of **36** by measuring the resistance reversing ability of the dibenzylmethylamine group. To determine whether the presence of **36** enhanced the potency of CQ, CQR parasites were incubated with a combination of CQ and **36** as well as CQ alone and **36** alone. This analysis illustrated that the activity of CQ did in fact increase when used in combination with **36** compared to the individual activity of CQ which suggests that the dibenzylmethylamine group is able to interact with the CQR PfCRT[74].

To corroborate this finding, the *X. laevis* oocyte PfCRT expression system was used to directly determine whether the dibenzylmethylamine group is a CQ-resistance reverser through its interaction with PfCRT. These experiments demonstrated that CQ transport into the oocyte cytosol by CQR PfCRT was inhibited in the presence of **36**. This observation is consistent with the results of the isobologram analysis and further confirms the CQ chemosensitising ability of **36**[63,73]. The mechanism of CQ efflux inhibition by **36** is unknown, but it is hypothesised that in CQR strains, the dibenzylmethylamine side chain binds and interacts with a greater affinity to the presumed CQ binding region of PfCRT compared to that of CQ which subsequently prevents the extrusion of CQ from the DV.

Compound **36** was evaluated for *in vivo* antimalarial efficacy in a *Plasmodium berghei*-infected murine model, and **36** was shown to reduce parasitaemia by 97% after a single oral administration of 30 mg/kg of **36** compared to the negative control[74]. Although **36** displayed promising antimalarial activity, there were difficulties in its developability due to potential toxicity issues that could arise specifically pertaining to systemic accumulation, due to its highly lipophilic nature, and possibly fatal cardiac arrhythmias as a result of human ether-a-go-go-related gene (hERG) channel binding, which is often associated with quinoline-based drugs[76].

1.7.2. Pyridodibemequines and their metabolites

Pyridodibemequines (PDBQs) are the next generation of DBQ derivatives which were designed to improve the physicochemical properties of the DBQ, specifically by reducing the lipophilicity of the compound to alleviate the potential systemic toxicity and cardiotoxicity risks. The terminal phenyl ring of the dibenzylmethylamine group of the DBQ was replaced with a pyridyl ring to produce a PDBQ. The introduction of the nitrogen atom on the aromatic ring is hypothesised to reduce the molecule's lipophilicity, and therefore, reduce hERG channel binding as well as systemic accumulation. Although the PDBQ compounds have not yet been investigated for their ability to inhibit transport of CQ by CQR PfCRT, they are hypothesised to interact with PfCRT in a comparable manner to the DBQs as both series display similar side chain structures[75]. Analogues of the PDBQ series are either chloro- or cyano-substituted at position 7 on the quinoline ring and additionally vary in the orientation of the modified dibenzylmethylamine side chain. A subset of analogues of this series, which were extensively investigated, are three chloro-substituted PDBQ compounds namely **49**, **43**, and **47** which are *ortho-*, *meta-*, and *para-*substituted, respectively as shown in **Figure 1.7**.

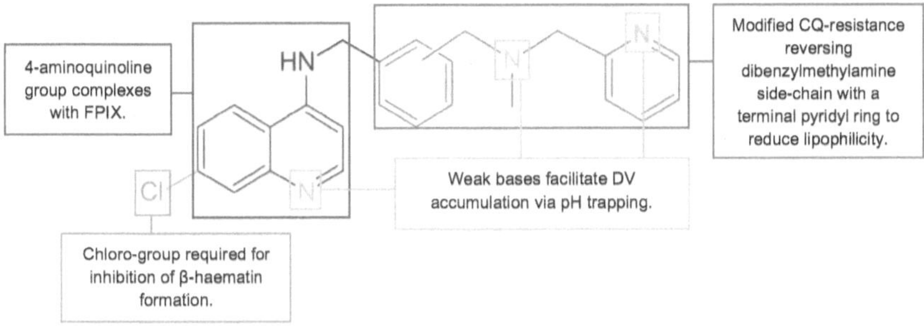

Figure 1.7. Proposed SAR of the resistance reversing PDBQs **49**, **43**, and **47** which are *ortho-*, *meta-*, and *para-* substituted, respectively[55,75].

Compounds **49**, **43**, and **47**, henceforth collectively referred to as the PDBQ parents, retained similar *in vitro* antimalarial activity against CQS parasites as compared to that of **36**. Additionally, the PDBQ parents were more active in a CQR strain of *P. falciparum* compared to the activity of CQ, which suggests dissimilar resistance mechanisms between CQ and the PDBQ compounds. In a *P. berghei*-infected murine model, the PDBQ parents displayed an 82–97% reduction in parasitaemia after oral compound administration of 30 mg/kg once a day for four days compared to the negative control. However, in a healthy murine model, it was shown that the *in vivo* oral absorption of these compounds was suboptimal[75]. Accordingly, it was unexpected that the PDBQ parents displayed favourable *in vivo* antimalarial efficacy given the low amount of intact drug that reached systemic circulation.

Metabolite identification studies were performed to elucidate the structures of any formed metabolites and to determine whether they retain any pharmacologically active groups, which could rationalise the observed *in vivo* efficacy in the *P. berghei*-infected murine model. The proposed metabolic pathway of the parent PDBQ is presented in **Figure 1.8**, and illustrates the formation of six different metabolites all of which are formed by cleavage at the nitrogen atom of the modified dibenzylmethylamine group, regardless of the orientation of the side chain[75].

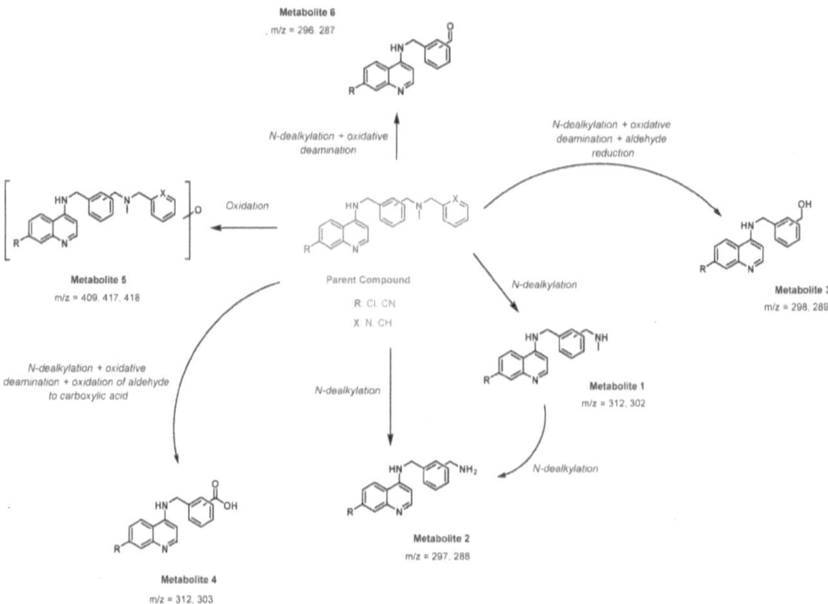

Figure 1.8. Proposed metabolic pathway of the PDBQ and DBQ parent compounds. Figure reproduced with permission from Joshi, M. C. *et al.* 4-Aminoquinoline Antimalarials Containing a Benzylmethylpyridylmethylamine Group are Active against Drug-Resistant *Plasmodium falciparum* and Exhibit Oral Activity in Mice. *Journal of Medicinal Chemistry* **60**, 10245-10256 (2017). Copyright (2017) American Chemical Society.

All PDBQ metabolites retained the 4-amino-7-chloroquinoline pharmacophore of the parent compound. Furthermore, metabolite 1 (M1) and metabolite 2 (M2) displayed the highest relative abundance compared to the other metabolites and are, therefore, regarded as the major metabolites which are proposed to be active against malaria[75]. Additionally, it is hypothesised that **36** produces similar major metabolites to **43** namely, **43M1** and **43M2**, which are suggested to account for the *in vivo* antimalarial efficacy of **36** in the *P. berghei*-infected murine model.

M1 and M2 of each parent PDBQ were synthesised to characterise the *in vitro* properties of the major metabolites and to evaluate whether they preserve the antimalarial activity of their parents. The *in vitro* antiplasmodial activity and cytotoxicity of the parents and major metabolites are indicated by the half-maximal inhibitory concentration (IC_{50}) value and are presented in **Table 1.1**. Indeed, M1 and M2 were shown to be pharmacologically active against various strains of *P. falciparum* which was anticipated since they conserve the 4-amino-7-chloroquinoline core of their parent. Moreover, this supports the hypothesis that the *in vivo* antimalarial activity of the PDBQ parents in the *P. berghei*-infected murine model was predominately attributed to these major metabolites. The *in vitro* antiplasmodial activities of the PDBQ parents in the CQS strain *Pf*NF54 ranged from 30–54 nM, and from 9–231 nM for the major metabolites. In the CQR strain *Pf*Dd2, the antiplasmodial activities of the PDBQ parents ranged from 124–151 nM, and that of the metabolites ranged from 51–953 nM[75,77]. In general, M1 displayed greater potency against the CQR strain relative to that of the PDBQ parents, M2, and CQ

The resistance index (RI) is the ratio of antiplasmodial activity between a drug-sensitive and drug-resistant strain, and relatively high values signify the presence of similar resistance mechanisms between drugs. The RI values of the PDBQ parents and metabolites against CQR *Pf*Dd2 ranged from 2–8, which suggests minimal cross-resistance with CQ[78].

The mammalian cytotoxicity of the PDBQ compounds was tested *in vitro* against a Chinese hamster ovarian (CHO) cell line[79]. Generally, all PDBQ parents and metabolites displayed minimal toxicity against the CHO cell line and were selective towards antiplasmodial activity; as denoted by the selectivity index (SI) which measures the specificity of drug action against the malaria parasite over mammalian cells. The hERG toxicity of the PDBQ parents and metabolites was also addressed as this was a high-risk factor for the developability of **36**. Prediction software suggested that the PDBQ parents could display slightly lower hERG channel binding compared to **36**. Furthermore, the major metabolites were predicted to demonstrate lower hERG liability compared to **36** and the PDBQ parents, potentially due to their relatively lower molecular weight[75,77,80]. A comprehensive evaluation of the *in vitro* absorption, distribution, metabolism, and excretion (ADME) of the PDBQ parents and metabolites is presented in **Chapter III, Section 3.1.3**.

Table 1.1. Summary of the *in vitro* antiplasmodial activities of the PDBQ parents and metabolites against CQS (*Pf*NF54 and *Pf*3D7) and CQR (*Pf*Dd2) strains of *P. falciparum* and their cytotoxicity against a mammalian cell line[74,75,77]

Compound	IC_{50} (nM)			RI[a]	Cytotoxicity	
	*Pf*NF54	*Pf*3D7	*Pf*Dd2		CHO IC_{50} (µM)	SI[b]
36	14	-[c]	26	2	10	660
49	54	61	137	3	40	740
49M1	10	9	51	5	11	1094
49M2	25	19	63	3	7	299
43	30	38	124	4	8	275
43M1	12	16	78	7	5	433
43M2	34	36	255	8	168	4984
47	39	33	151	4	16	408
47M1	9	13	55	6	6	617
47M2	231	291	953	4	14	58
CQ	8	14	226	28	36	4313

[a]RI= *Pf*Dd2 IC_{50}/*Pf*NF54 IC_{50}. [b]SI= CHO IC_{50}/*Pf*NF54 IC_{50}. [c]Data not available.

Due to their structural similarity to CQ, the mechanistic evaluation of the PDBQ parents and metabolites focused on the ability of these compounds to inhibit haemozoin formation. Using the cellular haem fractionation assay, the PDBQ parents and metabolites were shown to arrest the FPIX detoxification process thereby inhibiting haemozoin formation, which could be reflective of the activity of the 4-amino-7-chloroquinoline pharmacophore, as displayed in **Figure 1.9**[55,75,77]. It is conceivable that other unknown modes of action contributed to the observed antimalarial activity of the PDBQ parents and metabolites; however, it appears that haemozoin inhibition is the primary mechanism of action. Differences in the antiplasmodial activities of the *ortho-*, *meta-*, and *para-*orientated parents and metabolites are presumed to result from variabilities in their affinity towards the drug target and differential DV accumulation.

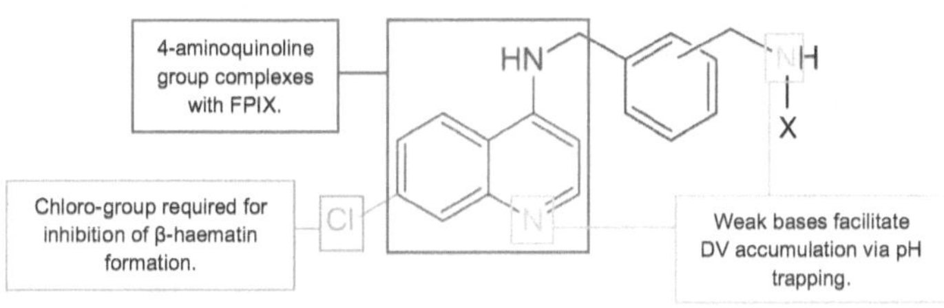

Figure 1.9. Proposed SAR of the major PDBQ metabolites **M1** and **M2** of **49**, **43**, and **47** which are *ortho-*, *meta-*, and *para-*substituted, respectively[55,75,77].

Since a fragment of the modified dibenzylmethylamine side chain of the PDBQ parent is cleaved off during the formation of the major metabolites, it is unknown whether M1 and M2 are able to interact with PfCRT to such a degree which gives them the ability to reverse CQ resistance. It was previously reported that common structural features of CQ chemosensitisers are two hydrophobic aromatic rings and an alkyl side chain with a protonatable nitrogen atom which is usually a tertiary or secondary amine. This specific molecular configuration allows the molecule to bind with PfCRT in the same regions which are responsible for CQ resistance[81,82]. Since M1 and M2 share similar structural features to those previously mentioned, there is a possibility that these metabolites could interact with PfCRT, but it is unknown whether this association culminates in reversing CQ resistance.

1.10. Introduction to research project and rationale

As observed over the past decades, the recurring obstacle of drug resistance has significantly impeded disease control efforts and has highlighted the necessity for continual development of alternative therapies which can be readily deployed in the event of attrition or complete failure by the current first-line treatment. While it is important to explore novel molecular targets, there is still value in exploiting and optimising existing pharmacophores. Of particular interest is the 4-amino-7-chloroquinoline group of CQ which is responsible for arresting the FPIX crystallisation pathway. As previously demonstrated, the mechanism of CQ resistance is independent of its mode of action, therefore, designing drugs which incorporate the 4-amino-7-chloroquinoline scaffold is still viable as its biological target remains unchanged and, thus, still vulnerable even in resistant strains[64]. This provides a rationale for continuing to explore the PDBQ series of parents and major metabolites as potential antimalarial leads, which forms the foundation of the work presented in this study.

The PDBQ parents displayed favourable *in vivo* antimalarial efficacy in a *P. berghei*-infected murine model which is hypothesised to be attributed to the activity of the major metabolites. Consequently, the major metabolites, M1 and M2, were synthesised, and they were generally shown to be favourably active *in vitro* against strains of *P. falciparum* and, pertinently, did not share cross-resistance with CQ. Additionally, M1 and M2 displayed selectivity towards antiplasmodial activity, and preliminary evaluations suggest that they are expected to display minimal toxicity risks associated with systemic accumulation and hERG-channel inhibition[75,77]. In light of these encouraging findings, further exploration of the PDBQ major metabolites as preclinical antimalarial leads was proposed with the primary objective of determining whether the selected candidates are able to suppress parasitaemia in a malaria-infected murine model.

In order to rationally select early lead candidates from the series of PDBQ metabolites, an extensive characterisation of their *in vivo* pharmacokinetics (PK) in a healthy murine model was needed. The approach for the PK studies of the PDBQ metabolites was to administer the parent PDBQ and quantify the parent and the formation of M1 and M2, with the intention of assessing the contribution of the major metabolites to the efficacy of the parent. Additionally, each pre-synthesised major metabolite was administered to determine their individual PK profiles. This process provided a greater understanding of the oral absorption behaviour of the major metabolites and imparted insight into whether the parent should be administered to deliver the active metabolites or whether the metabolite should be directly administered. Following these investigations, the rationally-selected lead compounds progressed to the *in vivo* efficacy evaluation to determine their antimalarial activity and PK in a *P. falciparum*-infected murine model.

Drug resistance allows parasites to proliferate in the presence of treatment and propagation of these resistant strains severely compromises therapeutic efficacy. This challenge needs to be constantly addressed as the evolution of resistance is inherent due to drug selective pressure. Combination therapy, utilising drugs with distinct mechanisms of action, is implemented to evade the development of resistance, by reducing the selective pressure, as it is hypothesised that a parasite is unlikely to simultaneously develop resistance towards two unrelated drug targets[16]. This highlights the importance of exploring antimalarial combinations during preclinical drug development. For this reason, *in vitro* isobologram analyses were performed to probe the combination potential of the prioritised PDBQ lead compounds with already established antimalarials. Additionally, the CQ-resistance reversing potential of the PDBQ parents and metabolites have not yet been explored; hence their capability for chemosensitising CQR strains is unknown. Therefore, isobologram analyses with the lead PDBQ compounds and CQ were performed in a CQR strain to determine whether the PDBQ potentiates the activity of CQ. If the PDBQ compounds do not preserve the resistance reversing ability of the DBQs, they can still be developed for use in combination therapy as they were still favourably active against the CQR strain *Pf*Dd2. A major drawback to the CQ-resistance reversing approach of the DBQ and PDBQ compounds is that essentially both drugs are targeting the same biological pathway. It can, however, be argued that the mechanism of resistance is unrelated to the molecular target and therefore, this combination might not exert the same selective pressure as monotherapy. Nonetheless, implementation of CQ-resistance reversers should ideally occur in settings where CQ resistance is prevalent. Given these limitations, greater focus was placed on partnering the PDBQ compounds with drugs of alternative mechanisms of action to haemozoin inhibition.

1.11. Aims

The aim of this project was to assess the potential of the chloro-substituted PDBQ series of parents and major metabolites as preclinical antimalarial candidates by investigating their *in vivo* PK and efficacy in healthy and *P. falciparum*-infected murine models. In addition, the *in vitro* interactions of the prioritised lead PDBQ compounds were assessed for their ability to be used in synergistic antimalarial combination therapy or as a CQ-resistance reverser.

1.12. Objectives

The overall objectives of this study were:

i. To develop and partially validate a bioanalytical method for the quantification of the PDBQ parents and major metabolites in whole blood using high-performance liquid chromatography coupled with tandem mass spectrometry (HPLC-MS/MS).

ii. To determine the *in vivo* PK profiles of the PDBQ parents and major metabolites in a healthy murine model through oral and intravenous (IV) administrations of the parent and preformed metabolites, in order to rationally select promising compounds for further antimalarial evaluation.

iii. To determine the *in vivo* PK and antimalarial efficacy of selected lead PDBQ compounds in a *P. falciparum*-infected humanised murine model.

iv. To investigate the *in vitro* antimalarial interactions, through isobologram analyses, of the selected lead PDBQ compounds with clinically relevant antimalarials in order to identify potential synergistic combination partners. Additionally, to evaluate the CQ-resistance reversing potential of the selected PDBQ lead compounds.

CHAPTER II

BIOANALYTICAL METHOD DEVELOPMENT AND VALIDATION

2.1. INTRODUCTION

2.1.1. Chapter aims

This chapter describes the bioanalytical methods used for the quantification of the PDBQ compounds from whole blood using reversed-phase HPLC-MS/MS. These assays were developed and partially validated for their specific application in the *in vivo* PK studies of the PDBQ parents and major metabolites in healthy and malaria-infected mice.

2.1.2. Bioanalytical techniques

A bioanalytical method encompasses the set of procedures that are used for the analysis of a compound of interest or analyte, such as a drug or metabolite, in a specific biological matrix. The assay should be designed and optimised to suit its intended purpose, whether it be for use in, for example, PK or toxicokinetic studies. Many analytical techniques, such as HPLC-MS/MS, have been developed to qualitatively or quantitatively determine an analyte in complex matrices. HPLC-MS/MS is highly sensitive and selective and utilises two independent partitioning methods. High-performance liquid chromatography (HPLC) separates molecules based on their physicochemical properties, and mass spectrometry (MS) further separates and detects molecules based on their mass-to-charge ratio (m/z)[83].

2.1.2.1. Reversed-phase high-performance liquid chromatography

Chromatography is a technique employed to separate components in a mixture. Detector systems, using ultraviolet detection or MS, can be coupled to the HPLC instrument to allow identification and quantification of analytes from the HPLC separation. Reversed-phase HPLC separates molecules based on their hydrophobicity and uses a polar liquid mobile phase to transport molecules through a non-polar stationary phase. The stationary phase, or reversed-phase analytical column, is composed of a solid silica support to which molecules of varying hydrophobicity are chemically bonded. A conventional reversed-phase analytical column is composed of octadecyl carbon chains (C18) which are anchored to surface silanol groups. A continuous flow of mobile phase, which is composed of water and a miscible organic solvent, such as acetonitrile (ACN) or methanol (MeOH), is used to carry molecules through the stationary phase[84,85].

Water has the highest polarity followed by MeOH then ACN; therefore, in reversed-phase chromatography, ACN has the highest elution strength for non-polar compounds followed by MeOH then water, which is the weakest solvent of hydrophobic molecules[83,85]. Different ratios of the aqueous and organic phases alter the overall polarity of the solvent system. For example, a relatively high aqueous composition increases the polarity of the solvent system and thus promotes the solubility of hydrophilic molecules in the mobile phase, which causes them to be displaced from the non-polar stationary phase.

Constituents in a mixture selectively partition or adsorb between the mobile and stationary phases based on their physicochemical properties and their varying degrees of interaction with each phase. Neutral molecules with hydrophobic functional groups will display greater interaction with the non-polar stationary phase than the polar aqueous mobile phase and will, therefore, be retained on the column for longer. This can be compared to neutral molecules with hydrophilic functional groups which display less column retention as they exhibit greater affinity to the polar aqueous mobile phase than the non-polar stationary phase. After eluting from the column, the molecule travels with the HPLC eluent to the detection system[83,86].

Biological samples contain a broad range of structurally-diverse molecules, and often gradient elution is adopted to enhance the separation efficiency of components in complex matrices. With gradient chromatography, the composition of the mobile phase progressively increases to a high percentage of organic solvent. This gradual change in solvent polarity allows better separation of molecules, which expand a broad range of chemistries, as they are expected to demonstrate varied affinities to the stationary and mobile phases, causing them to elute at different times[87].

Reversed-phase HPLC is primarily applied to separate neutral molecules since ionised molecules generally display greater hydrophilic interaction with the polar mobile phase than the non-polar stationary phase and thus show weak column retention and poor separation. Additionally, charged molecules can display secondary interactions with the stationary phase, which can result in undesirable peak tailing[84]. The inclusion of mobile-phase pH modifiers can be used to suppress the ionisation of functional groups which can improve chromatography by increasing non-polar stationary-phase retention. For ion-suppression chromatography, selective pH control is adopted where the pH of the mobile phase should be 2 units below or 2 units above the negative logarithm of the acid disassociation constant (pK_a) of the weakly acidic or weakly basic ionisable functional group, respectively[84,88]. Due to the acidic nature of silica, it is important to keep the mobile phase within the working pH range of the analytical column to prevent degradation of the stationary phase silica support[84].

2.1.2.2. Mass spectrometry

MS identifies molecular ions based on their m/z and can, therefore, further separate components that co-elute from the HPLC system. The mechanism of molecular ion detection using MS is ordered by two separate techniques. The first occurs within the atmospheric pressure ionisation (API) interface of the MS, where the HPLC eluent is delivered. Within the API interface, electrospray ionisation (ESI) occurs where liquid-phase ions are converted to gas-phase ions. The second set of processes occurs within the high vacuum region of the mass analyser, where the formed gas-phase ions are sequentially filtered based on their m/z[89,90].

The following describes techniques and instrument setting terminologies specific to SCIEX mass analysers. HPLC eluent enters the API interface through an electrospray probe. A potential difference exists between the electrospray capillary tip and the entrance to the high vacuum mass analyser region, which allows the movement of charged molecules through the interface. ESI requires the analyte to be charged in solution prior to entering the API interface as molecules which are electrically neutral are unable to enter the mass analyser. As the sample flows through the metal capillary within the electrospray probe, high voltage, or IonSpray voltage, and nebulising gas (GS1) are applied to the liquid which creates an aerosol of highly charged droplets at the capillary tip. In the API interface, the droplet solvent rapidly evaporates with the application of drying gas (GS2) and additional heat provided by the GS2 temperature (TEM)[90]. As desolvation occurs, the droplet volume decreases, which subsequently increases the electrostatic repulsion between excess surface charges. When the surface charge repulsion exceeds the surface tension, the droplet explodes through Coulomb fission to produce smaller charged droplets. Continuous droplet desolvation, increase in surface charge density, and Coulomb fission produces very small, highly charged droplets. The ultimate generation of singular gas-phase ions can be explained by the ion evaporation model which suggests that a single ion can be emitted from the evaporating droplet when the radius of the droplet reaches 10 nm or less[91,92,93,94].

The ESI mode can either be positive or negative. When the detection of protonated analytes is required, the positive ion mode is used; where the electrospray capillary tip is positively charged, and the counter electrode is negatively charged. This allows the movement of positively charged ions through the API interface and into the mass analyser. The converse is true for the negative ion mode, which is used to detect negatively charged, deprotonated species. The predominant droplet surface charge is dependent on the ionisation mode; for example, in positive ion mode, excess positively charged ions will migrate to the droplet surface and undergo Coulomb fission more readily than negatively charged ions[90,94].

The API interface and the mass analyser region are partitioned by a curtain plate and an orifice plate which houses the sampling aperture. As singular gas-phase ions are produced, they are transferred through a potential difference to the sampling orifice. A counterflow of neutral curtain gas (CUR) blows outwards, between the curtain plate and the orifice plate, towards the incoming ions. This process assists in preventing solvent vapours and ambient air from entering the orifice, thereby protecting the mass analyser from contamination. In addition, a declustering potential (DP) is applied on the orifice plate, which prevents ions from aggregating[89,90].

SCIEX mass analysers use a series of quadrupoles, each composed of four symmetrically-arranged parallel, equidistant rods, which generate an electromagnetic field using radio frequency (RF) and direct current (DC). Ions travel through the central axis of the quadrupole, and the electromagnetic field can be controlled to selectively stabilise the trajectory of specific ions based on their m/z. The mass-filtering quadrupoles use RF and DC to stabilise ions of specific m/z values, whereas only RF is applied to guide ions through the non-mass filtering quadrupoles. When gas-phase ions pass through the sampling orifice, they enter into the high-vacuum region of the mass analyser into the first quadrupole, Q0. An entrance potential (EP) is applied to focus the ions in Q0 and guide them through, into the mass analyser. Ions from Q0 are transferred to the first mass-filtering region in quadrupole 1 (Q1) where the ionised analyte or precursor ion is stabilised based on its m/z. Ions which are not of the selected m/z display an unstable trajectory through the quadrupole and are removed from Q1[89,90]. Precursor ions of the selected m/z are accelerated into quadrupole 2 (Q2), or the collision cell, through the collision cell entrance potential (CEP). Within Q2, an inert gas, such as nitrogen, collides with the precursor ion and generates ion fragments in a reproducible manner. The degree of collision-induced dissociation of the precursor ion is determined by the applied collision energy (CE) as well as the collision gas (CAD) which controls the collision gas pressure within Q2[89,90]. A collision cell exit potential (CXP) is used to guide fragment ions out of Q2 and into quadrupole 3 (Q3) where they undergo the second mass filtering. In Q3, specific product ions of the fragmented precursor ion are stabilised, and those ions which are not selected are deflected out of Q3. The selected fragment ions are then detected using a detection system which converts the incident fragment ion energy into electrical signals and sends the response to the data acquisition system. The generated signal is proportional to the fragment ion intensity[89,90].

A triple quadrupole mass analyser, as described above, uses two separate mass filtering procedures, in Q1 and Q3, and is referred to as tandem mass spectrometry (MS/MS). MS/MS is highly specific and comprises the method of multiple reaction monitoring (MRM), where an analyte is monitored by selected unique transitions of its precursor ion to its specific product ions[90].

2.1.2.3. Sample preparation

Sample preparation techniques are primarily designed to remove biological matrix components which are unsuitable for HPLC-MS/MS analysis. Whole blood matrices are complex and consist of erythrocytes suspended in plasma and proteins. The presence of these macromolecules can interfere with the HPLC-MS/MS analysis by blocking the analytical column or the MS capillary needle and, therefore, need to be removed from the sample to ensure correct performance of the analytical method.

Protein precipitation is an extraction technique that is used to separate small molecules from the proteins in a biological matrix. Water-miscible organic solvents, such as ACN or MeOH, are used to aggregate and precipitate proteins in aqueous blood. Additionally, changes to the pH of the biological matrix can decrease the solubility of proteins and cause them to come out of solution. Conformational changes to the protein structure allow the protein-bound analyte to be released into the extraction solvent. Small molecules can then be isolated by removing the insoluble proteins from the sample through centrifugation. The analyte should be soluble in the extraction solvent to ensure favourable and consistent recovery[95,96,97]. The extraction procedure does not necessarily need to recover the total amount of analyte present in the sample; it is more important that the method is reproducible and consistent at high and low concentrations[98]. A drawback to protein precipitation is that it is a relatively crude and non-selective sample preparation technique and, as a result, numerous other nonprotein matrix contaminants, such as phospholipids and fatty acids, can remain in solution with the analyte. Therefore, during the bioanalytical method validation procedure, the influence of endogenous matrix components on analyte detection should be addressed[99,100].

2.1.3. Method validation

Following the development of the HPLC-MS/MS and sample preparation methods, the assay is validated to ensure that it is optimised and suitable for its intended application. The validation procedure addresses the analyte recovery from the biological matrix, matrix effects, selectivity, sensitivity, accuracy, and precision as well as analyte stability throughout the assay conditions. A successful bioanalytical method validation which demonstrates assay accuracy and precision ensures the generation of reliable quantitative HPLC-MS/MS data. The bioanalytical methods presented in this chapter were developed and partially validated based on the fit-for-purpose concept, generally used for preclinical studies, as recommended in the guidelines published by the United States (US) Food and Drug Administration and the European Medicines Agency[98,101].

2.1.3.1. Calibration curve

A calibration curve is used to determine the unknown analyte concentration in study samples. A range of calibration standards are used to assign a specific known concentration to an instrument response or analyte peak area. The unknown analyte concentration in the experimental sample can be determined from the calibration curve by comparing the instrument response of the unknown concentration to the instrument responses of the known concentrations. A linear or quadratic regression model, with or without weighting, is often used to define the relationship between analyte concentration, on the x-axis, and instrument response, on the y-axis, which is reported as the internal standard (ISTD)-normalised analyte peak area. The calibration curve should ideally be within the linear, dynamic range of the MS, however, at higher analyte concentrations, ion source or detector saturation can occur which results in a non-linear response, depicted by the curvature of the regression line. The simplest regression model, which best fits the data, should be used to describe the relationship between concentration and instrument response. The correlation coefficient (r) parameter is used to evaluate the fit of the regression where an r value close to 1 indicates a strong, positive relationship between analyte concentration and instrument response[102].

Reference standards of known concentration are used to generate the calibration curve, and quality control (QC) samples, also of known concentration, are quantified against the calibration curve to monitor the performance and reliability of the assay in determining unknown experimental concentrations. Calibration standard and QC samples are prepared by spiking known concentrations of analyte into double blank matrix, which is free of analyte and ISTD. The double blank biological matrix should be similar in composition to that of the experimental samples to ensure consistent analyte recovery and HPLC-MS/MS detection of all reference and study samples[102].

The calibration curve is bound by the upper limit of quantification (ULOQ) and the lower limit of quantification (LLOQ). The calibration curve should include at least 6 non-zero reference standards, as well as the blank which is processed with ISTD and contains zero analyte, and the double blank which is processed without ISTD and also contains zero analyte. QC samples should be prepared to concentrations which test the assay accuracy and precision over the entire calibration range. The high quality control (HQC) should be approximately 75% of the ULOQ, the medium QC should be midrange, and the low quality control (LQC) should be within 3 times the LLOQ. The analytical range should reflect the expected concentration range of the experimental study samples[98,101,102].

2.1.3.2. Internal standard

An ISTD is a compound that is used to compensate for variability in the sample preparation procedure as well as normalise differential instrument response which could be due to, for example, variable sample injection volumes and matrix effects. The ISTD should be a structural analogue of the analyte or preferably, if available, a stable isotopically labelled analyte; this ensures that they both behave similarly during the bioanalytical procedure. The ISTD is added at equal concentration to all calibration standard, QC, and experimental samples at the earliest possible stage of sample preparation. Normalising the analyte response with the ISTD response will improve the accuracy and precision of the bioanalytical method[103,104].

2.1.3.3. Accuracy

Accuracy describes the closeness of the back-calculated concentration value, obtained by the bioanalytical method, to its nominal concentration value. To demonstrate acceptable accuracy, the assay determined concentration values of the calibration standard and QC samples should not deviate by more than ± 15% of their nominal concentration, and in the case of the LLOQ and LQC, the accuracy should be within ± 20% of the nominal concentration[98,101].

2.1.3.4. Precision

Precision measures the degree of assay reproducibility at each concentration level and describes how close the back-calculated concentration values are to one another. Precision is measured using two or more replicates for each concentration level of standard and QC samples. The precision at each concentration level is statistically calculated and expressed as the percentage coefficient of variation (CV). For acceptable bioanalytical assay precision, the CV value at each standard and QC concentration level should not exceed 15%, except for the LLOQ and LQC where the CV should not exceed 20%[98,101].

2.1.3.5. Selectivity

Selectivity is defined as the ability of the bioanalytical method to differentiate the analyte and ISTD from other endogenous matrix components present in the sample. The selectivity of an assay is determined by evaluating for interferences at the expected retention time (R_T) of the analyte or ISTD in double blank matrix. Acceptable assay selectivity is demonstrated when the response of interfering components in the double blank is ≤ 20% of the analyte response in the LLOQ, and for the ISTD the response in the double blank should be ≤ 5% of the ISTD response in the LLOQ. A selective HPLC-MS/MS method ensures that the analyte is quantified with adequate accuracy and precision[98,101].

2.1.3.6. Sensitivity

The sensitivity of the bioanalytical method, as described by the LLOQ, is the lowest concentration of analyte that can be reliably quantified with acceptable accuracy, between 80–120%, and acceptable precision of ≤ 20%. In addition, the analyte response in the LLOQ should be 5 times greater than the analyte response in the double blank; this can be evaluated by determining the analyte signal-to-background noise ratio (S/N), which should be ≥ 5[98,101].

2.1.3.7. Acceptance criteria for an analytical batch

An analytical batch is analysed in one continuous run and includes the calibration standards, QC samples, blank, and double blank samples and, if applicable, the experimental study samples. The reliability and acceptance of the assay determined concentration data is dependent on whether the calibration standard and QC samples are quantified within their predefined limits of accuracy and precision, as discussed in **Section 2.1.3.3** and **Section 2.1.3.4**. Additionally, at least 75% of the calibration standards, including the LLOQ and ULOQ, and at least 67% of the QC samples should acceptably pass. Furthermore, at least 50% of the replicates at each concentration level should fulfil the accuracy and precision acceptance criteria[98,101].

2.1.3.8. Carryover

Carryover refers to the transfer of analyte from a previously injected sample to the subsequent sample. This could occur as a result of the analyte adsorbing onto components of the HPLC injection system and then being introduced in the analysis of the next sample. Additionally, analytes which are strongly retained on the analytical column or those which display secondary interactions with the stationary phase can also display carryover effects, especially at higher analyte concentrations. Carryover should be minimised as it affects the sensitivity, accuracy, and precision of the bioanalytical method, particularly at the lower concentration range of the calibration curve[105]. Analyte carryover is evaluated by determining the transfer of analyte from the ULOQ to the blank, and ISTD carryover is assessed by the transfer of ISTD from the blank to the double blank. Acceptable carryover is demonstrated when the analyte response in the blank is $\leq$ 20% of the analyte response in the LLOQ; and the ISTD response in the double blank should be $\leq$ 5% of the ISTD response in the LLOQ[98,101].

2.1.3.9. Matrix effects

A matrix effect arises when co-eluting endogenous matrix components interfere with the ESI mechanism of the analyte, which ultimately alters the efficiency of gas-phase ion production. This can be demonstrated by ion suppression where a reduction in analyte response is observed or as ion enhancement which is indicated by an increase in analyte response. Although the actual mechanism of ion suppression is unknown, one theory suggests that this effect occurs as a result of charged matrix components which compete with the analyte for the droplet surface. Additionally, it has been proposed that the presence of less volatile solutes can alter the efficiency of droplet formation or evaporation during ESI, which results in a reduction of analyte gas-phase ion production[106,107]. Alternatively, background ions can enhance the formation of analyte gas-phase ions thereby increasing the analyte signal[107,108].

Matrix effects should be assessed during validation as it can affect the accuracy and precision of the bioanalytical method as well as compromise assay sensitivity and selectivity. The sample preparation procedure and chromatographic separation method should be optimised to minimise matrix effects. The matrix factor (MF) can be used to quantitatively evaluate the presence and extent of any matrix effect. The MF is the ratio of the analyte response in a post-extraction spiked matrix to the analyte response, at the same concentration, in a matrix-free solution. An MF value less than 1 or greater than 1 indicates ion suppression or ion enhancement, respectively, and an MF value equal to 1 indicates that the sample matrix does not contribute to the ionisation process of the analyte[101,109]. The ISTD is used to correct for matrix effects; therefore, in addition to having similar ionisation properties, the analyte and the ISTD should have similar elution times to allow them to encounter comparable matrix effects.

2.1.3.10. Analyte stability

Stability is assessed to determine whether the analyte is susceptible to degradation during the bioanalytical procedure; this could be as a result of chemical, physical, or metabolic processes. Analyte instability will challenge the accuracy and precision of the assay as well as the reliability of the generated quantification data. The stability of an analyte is expressed as a percentage of the reference where the analyte response under the test condition is compared to the analyte response of the reference sample, which represents a relative complete response. Acceptable stability is demonstrated when the analyte response under the test condition does not deviate by more than 15% from the response of the reference value. When high instability is demonstrated, further investigations should be performed to determine the cause, and the bioanalytical method should be revised to overcome analyte degradation by, for example, changing the storage conditions or using an antioxidant[98,101,110,111].

2.2.4. Pyridodibemequine parent and metabolite analytical chemistry

Bioanalytical assays were developed and partially validated for the quantification of the PDQB compounds and the ISTD from whole blood. The PDBQ compound, **126**, was used as an ISTD for all analytes. Compound **126** is a structural analogue of the PDBQ parents and is cyano-substituted at position 7 on the quinoline ring, as shown in **Table 2.1**. The first series of bioanalytical assays, as described in **Section 2.3.1**, were developed for the PK studies of the PDBQ parents and major metabolites in healthy mice, as presented in **Chapter III**. In addition to investigating the PK of the preformed major metabolites, these studies also evaluated the formation of the major metabolites after administration of the parent PDBQ. As a result, the HPLC-MS/MS methods, for each *ortho-*, *meta-*, and *para-* set of compounds, were developed to simultaneously detect and quantify the parent PDBQ, M1, M2, and the ISTD, as shown in **Table 2.1**.

The second series of bioanalytical assays, as described in **Section 2.3.2**, were developed for the PK studies of the lead PDBQ candidates, **43M1** and **47M1**, in malaria-infected mice, as presented in **Chapter IV**. Only the preformed metabolite was administered for these studies; therefore, the HPLC-MS/MS methods were developed to detect only the administered compound. **Table 2.1** displays the analytical chemistry of the ISTD and the PDBQ parents and metabolites and includes each compound's predicted pK_a values which were determined using MarvinSketch software version 18.20.0 (ChemAxon, Budapest, Hungary).

Table 2.1. Molecular structure, chemical formula, molecular weight, purity, and predicted pKa values of the PDBQ series of compounds

Analyte		Molecular structure	Chemical formula	Exact mass (Da)	HPLC purity (%)	pK_a 1	pK_a 2	pK_a 3
ISTD	**126**	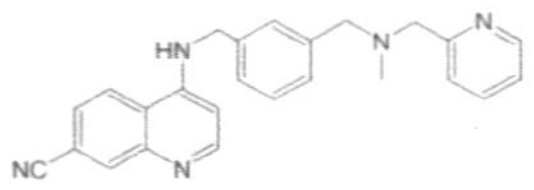	$C_{25}H_{23}N_5$	393.2	99.5	2.28	7.61	2.88
SET 49 *ortho-*	**49**	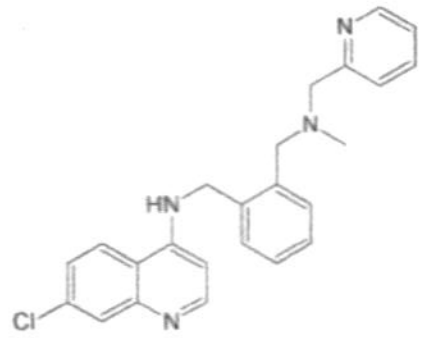	$C_{24}H_{23}ClN_4$	402.1	97.7	7.11	7.79	2.61
	49M1	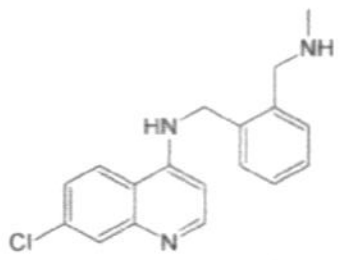	$C_{18}H_{18}ClN_3$	311.1	95.3	7.27	9.34	-
	49M2	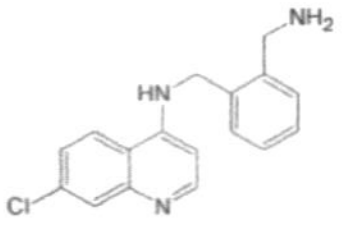	$C_{17}H_{16}ClN_3$	297. 1	95.2	7.27	9.22	-

Table 2.1. (continued)

Analyte		Molecular structure	Chemical formula	Exact mass (Da)	HPLC purity (%)	pK_a 1	pK_a 2	pK_a 3
	43	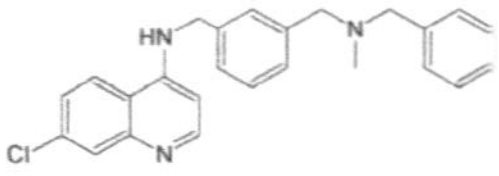	$C_{24}H_{23}ClN_4$	402.1	98.3	7.11	7.77	2.58
SET 43 *meta-*	**43M1**	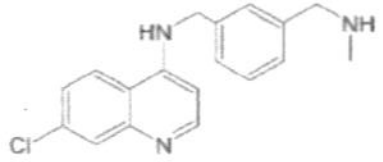	$C_{18}H_{18}ClN_3$	311.1	91.0	7.27	9.36	-
	43M2	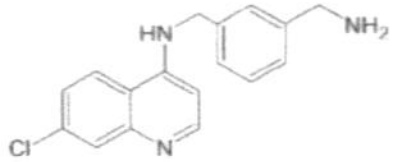	$C_{17}H_{16}ClN_3$	297. 1	96.3	7.27	9.27	-
	47	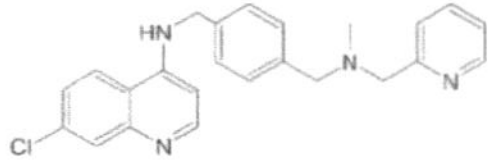	$C_{24}H_{23}ClN_4$	402.1	98.6	7.11	7.78	2.58
SET 47 *para-*	**47M1**	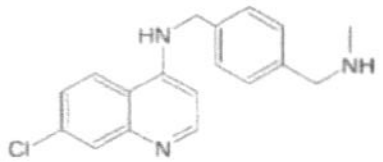	$C_{18}H_{18}ClN_3$	311.1	95.9	7.27	9.37	-
	47M2	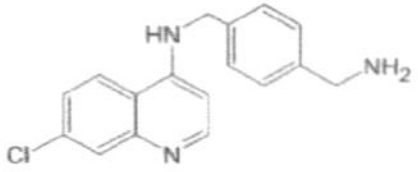	$C_{17}H_{16}ClN_3$	297. 1	98.0	7.27	9.29	-

2.2. METHODS

2.2.1. Materials

The PDBQ parent and metabolite compounds were synthesised at the Department of Chemistry, University of Cape Town (UCT). The HPLC purity of the compounds is presented in **Table 2.1**. The water (H_2O) used was purified by a Millipore Elix 10 reverse osmosis and Milli-Q® Gradient A 10 polishing system (Millipore, Massachusetts, US). The chemicals and reagents used for the bioanalytical methods were HPLC-MS grade and are presented in **Table 2.2**. **Table 2.3** presents the chemicals and reagents used for the PK dosing vehicle stability assessments.

Table 2.2. List of HPLC-MS grade materials used for the bioanalytical methods and the suppliers from which they were purchased

Material	Supplier
25% (v/v) ammonium hydroxide (NH_4OH) solution	Sigma-Aldrich (Merck, Missouri, US)
ACN	Honeywell (Burdick & Jackson, Michigan, US)
Dimethyl sulfoxide (DMSO)	Sigma-Aldrich
Formic acid (FA)	Sigma-Aldrich
MeOH	Honeywell

Table 2.3. List of materials used for the oral and IV dosing vehicles for the PK studies in healthy and malaria-infected mice and the suppliers from which they were purchased

Material	Supplier
Ethanol (EtOH)	Honeywell
Hydroxypropyl methylcellulose (HPMC)	Sigma-Aldrich
N,N-Dimethylacetamide (DMA)	Sigma-Aldrich
Polyethylene glycol 400 (PEG400)	Sigma-Aldrich
Polypropylene glycol (PPG)	Sigma-Aldrich
Tween80®	Sigma-Aldrich

The biological matrix obtained from the PK studies in healthy mice was murine whole blood. Native murine whole blood was obtained from the Medical School Animal Unit, UCT. The matrix collected from the PK studies in malaria-infected mice was humanised murine whole blood which consisted of a ratio of 1:1 of murine to human erythrocytes. Native humanised murine whole blood was collected from the Drug Discovery and Development Centre (H3D) animal unit, Division of Clinical Pharmacology, UCT. Ethical clearance was granted by the Animal Ethics Committee of the Faculty of Health Sciences (FHS), UCT. The ethics reference numbers are 013/028, 017/026, and 017/025. Lithium heparin anticoagulant was consistently used for all PK studies and bioanalytical assays. The composition of each biological matrix is hypothesised to be similar between batches as all mice are identical in genetics, age, diet, and environment.

2.2.2. Instrumentation

Analyte detection (MS/MS) was performed using a series of SCIEX triple quadrupole MS systems, namely an API 2000, API 3200, and API 5500 (SCIEX, Toronto, Canada). All instruments were equipped with a TurboIonSpray® probe for ESI. To achieve chromatography, the API 2000 and API 3200 were each coupled to an Agilent 1100 Series HPLC system, and the API 5500 was coupled to an Agilent 1260 Infinity II HPLC system (Agilent Technologies, California, US). All HPLC systems included a binary pump, autosampler, and column oven. Data acquisition and processing were achieved using

Analyst software version 1.5.2 for the API 2000 and API 3200, and version 1.6.3 for the API 5500 (SCIEX, Toronto, Canada).

2.2.3. Bioanalytical method development

2.2.3.1. Mass spectrometry

Analyte and ISTD MS detection was achieved by infusing a pure, standard solution of the compound into the instrument. The infusion concentration varied and was dependent on the sensitivity of each instrument. Analyte ionisation was investigated in acidic and basic infusion solutions with ACN or MeOH. The conditions which resulted in the most favourable ESI response was used for the final HPLC-MS/MS method. First, an initial manual tuning was carried out to verify the molecular weight of the precursor ion. Then the compound optimisation was performed to determine the product ion m/z values and the optimal ion source and gas detection parameters for each transition. The final MRM method included the product ion which displayed the highest relative intensity. The acquisition duration for each transition, or the dwell time, was set to allow sufficient data point collection.

2.2.3.2. Reversed-phase chromatography

Given the complex matrix of whole blood, a linear gradient elution method was developed to separate the analytes from matrix components. HPLC method development involved systematically optimising the following conditions to achieve acceptable peak shape and resolution: the organic mobile phase, the aqueous and organic starting conditions, the steepness of the gradient method, the flow rate, and the injection volume. Chromatography was optimised to ensure that the analyte did not elute at the solvent front with any unretained, polar molecules. Additionally, analyte elution was prevented during the column equilibration phase. Before use, mobile phases were degassed to remove dissolved air by sonication and helium sparging.

2.2.3.3. Sample preparation

The protein precipitation extraction method was developed and optimised at high and low concentrations which corresponded to each analyte's HQC and LQC concentration, as shown in **Table 2.4** and **Table 2.5**. Different extraction solvents, either MeOH or ACN, with or without an acid or base, were tested. The protein precipitant which yielded the most favourable and reproducible analyte recovery was chosen as the final extraction solvent.

The extraction efficiency of the final sample preparation procedure, as shown in **Section 2.3.1.3** and **Section 2.3.2.3**, was tested at each analyte's HQC and LQC concentration. The absolute recovery was determined by comparing the analyte response in the pre-extraction spiked matrix to the analyte response, at the same concentration, in the post-extraction spiked matrix, as shown in **Equation 2.1**. Pre-extraction spiked matrix samples were prepared by spiking HQC and LQC working solutions into whole blood, as described in **Section 2.2.4.1**. The post-extraction spiked matrix samples were prepared by extracting double blank whole blood with the relevant sample preparation procedure. The extracted supernatant was then spiked with the HQC and LQC working solutions to give the same final concentration as the pre-extraction matrix samples. The post-extraction spiked matrix compensates for matrix effects and, therefore, represents complete recovery. Pre-extraction and post-extraction spiked samples were processed according to the relevant extraction procedure, and then samples were submitted for HPLC-MS/MS analysis.

$$\text{Absolute recovery (\%)} = \frac{\text{ISTD-normalised analyte peak area of pre-extraction spiked matrix}}{\text{ISTD-normalised analyte peak area of post-extraction spiked matrix}} \times 100 \qquad \textbf{Equation 2.1}$$

2.2.4. Bioanalytical method validation

The method validation experiments to determine assay selectivity, sensitivity, accuracy, precision, and carryover were performed during the analytical run of each analyte's validation calibration curve. Standard, QC, blank, and double blank samples were prepared in either duplicate or triplicate.

Ultra-low temperature is often used for bioanalytical sample storage as small molecules are generally more stable at lower temperatures, as the rate of chemical and metabolic degradation is lower. It was hypothesised that the PDBQ series of compounds were stable in whole blood at -80°C, therefore, experimental and bioanalytical reference samples were stored at -80°C until use[111,112,113,114]. Additionally, the accuracy and precision of the calibration standard and QC samples were closely monitored during the validation phase to ensure that -80°C storage was suitable for the analytes.

Analyte stability was ascertained under the environmental and time conditions of the following procedures, calibration curve and QC preparation, sample preparation, PK dosing and experimental sampling, and HPLC MS/MS analysis. This included determining analyte stability in the stock solution, working solution, biological matrix, post-preparative solution, and PK dosing vehicles. Freeze-thaw stability was not assessed as all experimental samples were not refrozen or reprocessed after being thawed from -80°C.

2.2.4.1. Calibration curve

The calibration curve range for the PK studies in healthy mice was set to cover the concentration range typically observed in preclinical *in vivo* murine PK studies. Additionally, the LLOQ was determined based on the sensitivity of the MS/MS instrument. The calibration range for the PK studies in malaria-infected mice was determined using each compound's corresponding concentration data that was obtained from the PK studies in healthy mice.

Calibration standard, QC, and bioanalytical assay validation samples were prepared by parallel spiking working solutions into double blank whole blood, which matched the matrix of the PK study samples. The procedure was performed on ice unless otherwise indicated. The calibration standards and QCs were prepared independently from one another and used separate stock solutions. First, DMSO stock solutions were freshly prepared for each analyte. For the analytical methods that required the simultaneous quantification of the parent and two major metabolites, a calibration curve was prepared for each compound in the set by pooling all the analytes to the same starting concentration in a primary standard working solution (WS-), WS0, in ACN. The pooled analytes were then further diluted with ACN to prepare the first standard working solution or WS1. For the assays which required the quantification of only one metabolite, WS1 was prepared by directly diluting the analyte stock solution with ACN. All subsequent standard working solutions were made by serial dilutions with ACN to cover the relevant standard concentration range, as shown in

Table 2.4 and **Table 2.5**. The calibration standard samples were then prepared by spiking 4% (v/v) of the ACN working solution into an ambient-temperature whole blood aliquot. The sample was vortexed for 2 min and then left to equilibrate for 1 min at ambient temperature. Once all calibration standards were prepared, they were aliquoted and placed in storage at -80°C. The QC samples were then spiked using the same method as previously described for the preparation of the calibration standards.

Table 2.4 presents a general overview of the calibration standard and QC working solution concentrations, and the corresponding final whole blood concentrations that were used to construct the calibration curves for the PK analyses in healthy mice. As discussed in **Section 2.3.2.2**, for the PK studies in malaria-infected mice, the calibration curve was split to cover 2 different analytical ranges, as displayed in **Table 2.5**.

Table 2.4. Calibration standard and QC working solution concentrations and the corresponding whole blood concentrations used to construct the calibration curve for the PK analysis of the PDBQ compounds in healthy mice

	Working solutions in ACN		Standards and QCs in whole blood	
	Sample name	**Concentration (μg/ml)**	**Sample name**	**Concentration (ng/ml)**
	WS0[a]	200	-	-
	WS1	100	S1	4000
	WS2	75	S2	3000
	WS3	37.5	S3	1500
Standards	WS4	18.8	S4	750
	WS5	4.7	S5	187.5
	WS6	1.6	S6	62.5
	WS7	0.8	S7	31.3
	WS8	0.4	S8	15.6
	WS9	80	QC1 (HQC)	3200
QCs	WS10	40	QC2	1600
	WS11	2	QC3	80
	WS12	1	QC4 (LQC)	40

[a]W0 was only prepared to pool the parent, M1, and M2.

Table 2.5. Calibration standard and QC working solution concentrations and corresponding whole blood concentrations used to construct the calibration curve for the PK analysis of **43M1** and **47M1** in malaria-infected mice

	Calibration curve split	Working solutions in ACN		Standards and QCs in whole blood	
		Sample name	Concentration (μg/ml)	Sample name	Concentration (ng/ml)
Standards	Curve 1	WS1	150	S1	10000
	Curve 1	WS2	120	S2	8000
	Curve 1	WS3	90	S3	6000
	Curve 1 & 2	WS4	60	S4	4000
	Curve 1 & 2	WS5	30	S5	2000
	Curve 1 & 2	WS6	7.5	S6	500
	Curve 1 & 2	WS7	3.8	S7	250
	Curve 1 & 2	WS8	1.1	S8	75
	Curve 2	WS9	0.4	S9	25
	Curve 2	WS10	0.08	S10	5
	Curve 2	WS11	0.03	S11	2
QCs	Curve 1	WS12	110	QC1 (HQC)	7300
	Curve 1 & 2	WS13	45	QC2	3000
	Curve 1 & 2	WS14	15	QC3	1000
	Curve 1 & 2	WS15	1.5	QC4	100
	Curve 2	WS16	0.15	QC5	10
	Curve 2	WS17	0.06	QC6 (LQC)	4

Calibration curve samples were extracted in the same order of HPLC-MS/MS analysis, using the relevant sample preparation procedure, as described in **Section 2.3.1.3** and **Section 2.3.2.3**. Calibration standards, QCs, and blank matrix samples were run in either duplicate or triplicate. The analyte free blank and double blank matrix samples were processed with and without ISTD, respectively. Each replicate curve was sequentially injected in descending analyte concentration, except for the blank which was injected after the ULOQ and the double blank which was injected after the blank. When analysing PK study samples, each PK batch was run with its own calibration curve which was extracted concurrently with the PK samples. PK samples were positioned between the calibration curve samples in a non-randomised sequence.

Data processing was performed with Analyst software. Analyte and ISTD peak areas were automatically integrated, but each peak was manually inspected to ensure a consistent baseline. A standard calibration curve of ISTD-normalised analyte peak area (y-axis) against analyte concentration (x-axis) was generated. The best-fitting regression line was used to model the relationship between instrument response and concentration. The generated regression was used to back-calculate the concentrations of the QC and PK experimental study samples. The analytical run was either accepted or rejected based on the criteria outlined in **Section 2.1.3.7**.

2.2.4.2. Selectivity

To ascertain the assay selectivity, at least 4 aliquots of double blank whole blood matrix were extracted, without ISTD, according to the relevant sample preparation procedure, as described in **Section 2.3.1.3** and **Section 2.3.2.3**. The double blank samples were processed with the respective LLOQ sample. All samples were then submitted for HPLC-MS/MS analysis. The mean analyte and ISTD peak areas in the double blank and LLOQ samples were determined by Analyst software. The selectivity of the assay was numerically evaluated according to **Equation 2.2**. Additionally, double blank chromatograms were visually inspected for interference at the expected analyte retention time.

$$\text{Selectivity (\%)} = \frac{\begin{array}{c}\text{Analyte or ISTD} \\ \text{peak area in double blank}\end{array}}{\begin{array}{c}\text{Analyte or ISTD} \\ \text{peak area in LLOQ}\end{array}} \times 100 \qquad \textbf{Equation 2.2}$$

Acceptable assay selectivity was demonstrated when the calculated selectivity value is ≤ 20% for the analyte and ≤ 5% for the ISTD[98,101].

2.2.4.3. Sensitivity

To determine the assay sensitivity, two criteria had to be fulfilled for the LLOQ sample. First, the analyte peak area in the LLOQ had to be at least 5 times the analyte response in the double blank; this was numerically determined by the S/N value which had to be ≥ 5. Additionally, the LLOQ had to be quantified with acceptable accuracy and precision, as discussed in **Section 2.1.3.6**.

2.2.4.4. Carryover

Analyte carryover was assessed by injecting a blank matrix sample after the ULOQ and ISTD carryover was assessed by injecting a double blank matrix sample after the blank sample. The peak area in the relevant blank or double sample was compared to the respective peak area in the LLOQ sample, and the analyte carryover and ISTD carryover were calculated according to **Equation 2.3** and **Equation 2.4**, respectively.

$$\text{Analyte carryover (\%)} = \frac{\text{Analyte peak area in blank}}{\text{Analyte peak area in LLOQ}} \times 100$$ **Equation 2.3**

$$\text{ISTD carryover (\%)} = \frac{\text{ISTD peak area in double blank}}{\text{ISTD peak area in LLOQ}} \times 100$$ **Equation 2.4**

Acceptable analyte and ISTD carryover was demonstrated by carryover values $\leq 20\%$ and $\leq 5\%$ of the LLOQ, respectively[98,101].

2.2.4.5. Matrix effects

Matrix effects were assessed in each whole blood matrix with at least 4 replicates at each analyte's high and low concentration. ISTD matrix effects were tested at one value which corresponded to the ISTD concentration in the extraction solvent which was 300 ng/ml, 100 ng/ml, and 50 ng/ml for analysis on the API 2000, API 3200, and API 5500, respectively. For the bioanalytical assays used for the PK studies in healthy mice, the matrix effects were determined by pooling the analytes within each set. For the bioanalytical assays used for the PK studies in malaria-infected mice, the matrix effects were determined individually for each analyte. First, the matrix-free solutions were prepared by spiking analyte to HQC and LQC concentrations in 0.1% (v/v) NH_4OH in ACN. The post-extraction spiked matrix samples were prepared by extracting double blank whole blood, from at least 4 different lots, with the relevant sample preparation procedure, as described in **Section 2.3.1.3** and **Section 2.3.2.3**. The extracted supernatant was then spiked to the same HQC and LQC concentrations used for the matrix-free samples. The matrix-free and post-extraction spiked matrix samples were diluted with 0.1% (v/v) NH_4OH in ACN, using the same dilution volumes described in the sample preparation procedure. All samples were then submitted for HPLC-MS/MS analysis.

The MF was calculated according to **Equation 2.5**, which compares the analyte peak area in the presence of matrix components to the analyte peak area analysed with zero matrix effects. Additionally, the ISTD-normalised MF was calculated using **Equation 2.6**.

$$\text{MF} = \frac{\text{Analyte or ISTD peak area in post-extraction spiked matrix}}{\text{Analyte or ISTD peak area in matrix-free sample}}$$ **Equation 2.5**

$$\text{ISTD-normalised MF} = \frac{\text{Analyte MF}}{\text{ISTD MF}}$$ **Equation 2.6**

An MF value less than 1, greater than 1, or equal to 1 indicates ion suppression, ion enhancement, or no matrix effects, respectively[101]. The matrix effects had to be similar at the HQC and LQC concentrations to ensure consistent analyte ionisation along the calibration curve range.

2.2.4.6. Stock solution stability

To ascertain analyte stability during calibration curve standard and QC preparation, the analyte stock solution stability in DMSO for 1 h at ambient temperature was assessed. Two samples of analyte were weighed out; one was used as the reference and the other for the test condition. DMSO was added to the test condition sample to constitute a final concentration of 2 mg/ml. The test stock solution was then aliquoted at least 4 times, and the samples were left to stand at ambient temperature for 1 h. After 1 h, the reference samples were prepared by dissolving the test condition analyte with DMSO to a final concentration of 2 mg/ml. The test stock solution was then aliquoted at least 4 times. The test condition and reference sample aliquots were then diluted, using the same dilution steps, to a final concentration of 300 ng/ml. The first dilution was made with 0.1% (v/v) NH_4OH in ACN, which was spiked with the ISTD; and all subsequent dilutions were made with 0.1% (v/v) NH_4OH in ACN without ISTD. Samples were then submitted for LC-MS/MS analysis.

To determine the stability of the analyte, the ISTD-normalised analyte peak area under the test condition was compared to the ISTD-normalised analyte peak area of the reference, which represents complete stability, as displayed in **Equation 2.7**.

$$\text{Stability (\%)} = \frac{\text{ISTD-normalised analyte peak area in test condition}}{\text{ISTD-normalised analyte peak area in reference}} \times 100 \qquad \textbf{Equation 2.7}$$

The calculated stability of the test condition was required to be within the range of 85–100% of the reference value, and the methodology was revised if the observed analyte degradation exceeded 15%.

2.2.4.7. Working solution stability

To ascertain analyte stability during calibration curve standard and QC preparation, the analyte working solution stability in ACN for 1 h on ice was assessed. Working solution stability was determined by pooling the analytes within each set. The test samples and reference samples were prepared with at least 4 replicates at each HQC and LQC concentration. Two stock solution samples of the pooled analytes were freshly prepared before use, one for the reference and one for the test condition. The test stock solution sample was diluted with ACN to prepare working solutions at each HQC and LQC concentration. All test samples were placed on ice for 1 h. After 1 h, the reference stock solution was diluted with ACN to the same HQC and LQC concentrations of the test condition samples. All test condition and reference samples were diluted twofold with 0.1% (v/v) NH_4OH in ACN, which was spiked with ISTD. Samples were then submitted for HPLC-MS/MS analysis, and the percentage working solution stability was calculated according to **Equation 2.7**. The calculated stability of the test condition was required to be within the range of 85–100% of the reference value, and the methodology was revised if the observed analyte degradation exceeded 15%.

2.2.4.8. Bench-top biological matrix stability

To ascertain analyte stability during calibration curve standard and QC preparation, sample preparation and PK sampling, the analyte stability in whole blood for 1 h on ice was determined. The stabilities were assessed in each whole blood matrix with at least 4 replicates at each analyte's HQC and LQC concentration. For the bioanalytical assays used for the PK studies in healthy mice, the matrix stability was determined by pooling the analytes within each set. For the bioanalytical assays used for the PK studies in malaria-infected mice, the matrix stability was determined individually for each analyte. First, at least 12 aliquots each of HQC and LQC whole blood samples were prepared and stored at -80°C, as described in **Section 2.2.4.1**. On the day of analysis, at least 6 test condition aliquots of each HQC and LQC sample were removed from -80°C storage and placed on ice for 1 h. After 1 h, the remaining aliquots or reference samples were removed from -80°C storage and left to thaw on ice. All test condition and reference samples were then immediately extracted using the relevant sample preparation procedure as described in **Section 2.3.1.3** or **Section 2.3.2.3**. Samples were submitted for HPLC-MS/MS analysis, and the percentage matrix stability was calculated according to **Equation 2.7**. The calculated stability of the test condition was required to be within the range of 85–100% of the reference value, and the methodology was revised if the observed analyte degradation exceeded 15%.

2.2.4.9. Post-preparative stability

Post-preparative analyte stability was determined at ambient temperature for at least 24 h on-instrument, which covered the expected run time of the analytical batch. The stabilities were assessed in each whole blood matrix extract with at least 4 replicates at each analyte's HQC and LQC concentration. For the bioanalytical assays used for the PK studies in healthy mice, the on-instrument stability was determined by pooling the analytes within each set. For the bioanalytical assays used for the PK studies in malaria-infected mice, the on-instrument stability was determined individually for each analyte. HQC and LQC matrix samples were extracted according to the relevant sample preparation procedure, as described in **Section 2.3.1.3** or **Section 2.3.2.3**. All samples were submitted for HPLC-MS/MS analysis and then 24 h after the initial run, all samples were reinjected for analysis. The percentage post-preparative stability was calculated according to **Equation 2.7**. The calculated stability of the test condition was required to be within the range of 85–100% of the reference value, and the methodology was revised if the observed analyte degradation exceeded 15%.

2.2.4.10. Dosing vehicle stability

The oral and IV stabilities of the analyte in the respective dosing formulations were determined for 1 h on ice. The analyte was prepared in the oral formulation of 0.5% (w/v) HPMC in H_2O with 0.2% (v/v) Tween80®; the sample was vortexed and sonicated to ensure a homogenous particle suspension. Additionally, the IV sample was prepared by dissolving the analyte with the IV formulation of DMA:PPG:EtOH:PEG400 (5:24:6:15, v/v). Each formulation was prepared to a final concentration of 0.5 mg/ml, and all samples were stored on ice. Reference samples were taken in triplicate immediately after each formulation was prepared. The reference samples were diluted to a final concentration of 300 ng/ml with 0.1% (v/v) NH_4OH in ACN; the first dilution was made with ACN spiked with ISTD, and all subsequent dilutions were made with ISTD-free 0.1% (v/v) NH_4OH in ACN. After 1 h on ice, the test condition samples were taken in triplicate and diluted with the same procedure used to prepare the reference samples. All samples were submitted for HPLC-MS/MS analysis. The percentage stability in each dosing vehicle was calculated according to **Equation 2.7**. The calculated stability of the test condition was required to be within the range of 85–100% of the reference value, and the methodology was revised if the observed analyte degradation exceeded 15%.

2.3. RESULTS AND DISCUSSION

The bioanalytical method development and partial validation for the PDBQ compounds is presented in **Section 2.3.1** for the PK studies in healthy mice and in **Section 2.3.2** for the PK studies in malaria-infected mice. In instances where the results were similar or repetitive, such as those displayed by mass spectra, chromatograms, and calibration curves, only a representative figure is shown.

2.3.1. Bioanalytical method development and partial validation for the pharmacokinetic studies in healthy mice

The bioanalytical assays used for the PK studies in healthy mice, as presented in **Chapter III**, is described in this section. HPLC-MS/MS methods were developed to simultaneously detect the parent PDBQ, M1, M2, and the ISTD, **126**, in murine whole blood. The HPLC-MS/MS methods were partially validated for each analyte within each set of compounds. The HPLC-MS/MS assays for the quantification of the analytes in Set **49**, Set **43**, and Set **47** were developed and partially validated on the API 2000. Due to instrument capacity and scheduling, an additional HPLC-MS/MS method was developed for Set **43** on the API 3200; and partially validated to address selectivity, sensitivity, carryover, accuracy, precision, and matrix effects.

2.3.1.1. Mass spectrometry

All PDBQ compounds were monitored at unit resolution in the positive MRM mode. All analytes were infused in a solution of 0.1% (v/v) NH_4OH in ACN. A representative product ion mass spectrum of **47M1** is displayed in **Figure 2.1**. The parent ion [**47M1** + H]$^+$ was detected at m/z 312, and the most intense fragment ion was observed at m/z 105.

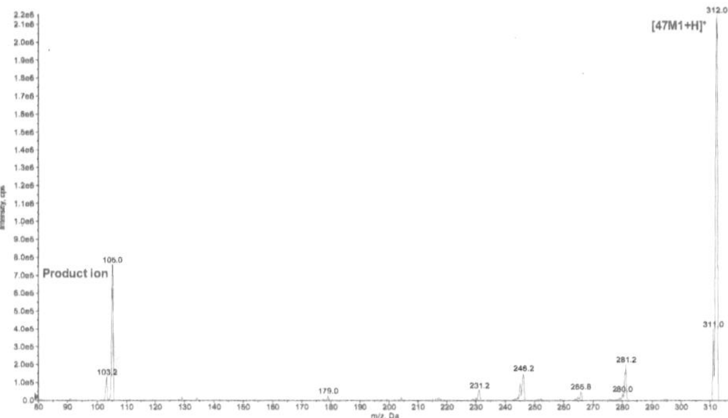

Figure 2.1. Product ion spectrum of **47M1** displaying [**47M1** + H]$^+$ at m/z 312 and the product ion fragments with the most intense peak at m/z 105.

The final MRM method for each analyte is presented in **Table 2.6** and **Table 2.7** for detection on the API 2000, and in **Table 2.8** and **Table 2.9** for detection of Set **43** on the API 3200. The tables display each analyte's protonated precursor ion to product ion m/z transition and the compound- and source-dependent parameters that were used for their detection.

Table 2.6. Source and gas parameter settings used for the detection of the analytes in Set **49**, Set **43**, and Set **47** on the API 2000

MS setting	Value
Ionisation mode	Positive
IonSpray voltage (V)	3000
TEM (°C)	450
GS1 (psi)	70
GS2 (psi)	70
CUR (psi)	30
CAD (psi)	7

Table 2.7. Compound-dependent parameter settings used for the detection of the analytes in Set **49**, Set **43**, and Set **47** on the API 2000

Analyte		Precursor ion (m/z)	Product ion (m/z)	Dwell time (ms)	DP (V)	EP (V)	CEP (V)	CE (eV)	CXP (V)
Set **49**	**49**	403.1	225.2	150	60	8	17	30	6
	49M1	312.1	105.2	150	40	9	23	50	2
	49M2	298.1	179.1	150	40	9	25	30	2
	126	394.2	105.1	150	60	8	17	50	2
Set **43**	**43**	403.1	105.2	150	30	9	19	40	2
	43M1	312.1	105.2	150	30	10	23	40	2
	43M2	298.1	120.2	150	30	9	17	40	2
	126	394.2	105.1	150	60	8	17	50	2
Set **47**	**47**	403.1	133.1	150	45	12	21	40	2
	47M1	312.1	134.1	150	60	9	15	30	2
	47M2	298.0	120.1	150	50	8	15	40	2
	126	394.2	105.1	150	60	8	17	50	2

Table 2.8. Source and gas parameter settings used for the detection of the analytes in Set **43** on the API 3200

MS setting	Value
Ionisation mode	Positive
IonSpray voltage (V)	5500
TEM (°C)	450
GS1 (psi)	50
GS2 (psi)	50
CUR (psi)	30
CAD (psi)	5

Table 2.9. Compound-dependent parameter settings used for the detection of the analytes in Set **43** on the API 3200

Analyte		Precursor ion (m/z)	Product ion (m/z)	Dwell time (ms)	DP (V)	EP (V)	CEP (V)	CE (eV)	CXP (V)
SET **43**	**43**	403.3	105.2	150	56	8	22	47	6
	43M1	312.3	105.0	150	46	7	20	43	4
	43M2	298.2	120.1	150	46	6	22	37	4
	126	394.3	105.2	150	51	6	22	45	4

2.3.1.2. Chromatography

Due to the ionisable amino functional groups of the PDBQ compounds, ion-suppression chromatography was employed. A basic mobile phase pH modifier was used to increase analyte retention on the non-polar analytical column and enhance peak shape. Despite the analytes being neutral under the ion suppression conditions of the highly basic HPLC mobile phase, they still displayed favourable detection in the positive ion mode using ESI, as shown in **Figure 2.1**. This observation is hypothesised to be attributed to a significant pH change of the HPLC eluent at the electrospray capillary, as well as a change in droplet pH during desolvation which effectively resulted in protonation of the analyte during ESI[115,116].

Chromatography of the analytes in Set **49**, Set **43**, and Set **47** was performed on an Agilent 1100 Series HPLC system using the same method as described here. Reversed-phase chromatographic separation of the parent PDBQ, M1, M2, and the ISTD was achieved using a Gemini-NX C18 110 Å (50 mm x 2 mm, 5 μM) analytical column (Phenomenex, California, US). On a normal analytical column, the weakly acidic silica support starts to solubilise when exposed to highly basic pH environments above 8[83]. Therefore, the Gemini-NX column was chosen as its silica support is highly stabilised and reinforced to allow it to resist degradation in extreme pH environments[117]. The mobile phase was delivered at a constant flow rate of 600 μl/min, and a gradient elution method was used, as outlined in **Figure 2.2**, with 0.1% (v/v) NH_4OH in H_2O (pH 10) (aqueous mobile phase) and 0.1% (v/v) NH_4OH in ACN (pH 10) (organic mobile phase). A post-column HPLC eluent flow split of 1:5 of instrument to waste was used to reduce liquid flow into the MS interface.

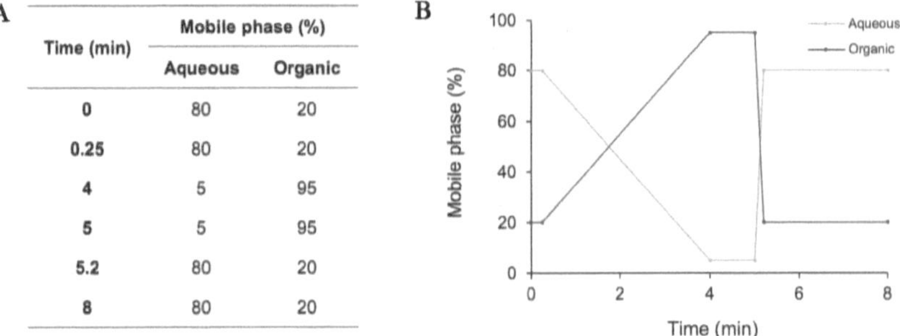

A

Time (min)	Mobile phase (%)	
	Aqueous	Organic
0	80	20
0.25	80	20
4	5	95
5	5	95
5.2	80	20
8	80	20

Figure 2.2. A HPLC gradient method and **B** graphical representation of the gradient method used for the separation of the parent PDBQ, its metabolites M1 and M2, and the ISTD.

Samples were housed in the autosampler at ambient temperature and were injected onto the column with an injection volume of 15 μl for detection on the API 2000 and 6 μl for detection on the API 3200. A needle wash with ACN was performed between injections. In addition, to further reduce carryover on the API 3200, a blank ACN column wash was performed between injections, using the HPLC gradient method described in **Figure 2.2.** A representative chromatogram of the analytes in Set **47** is presented in **Figure 2.3.**

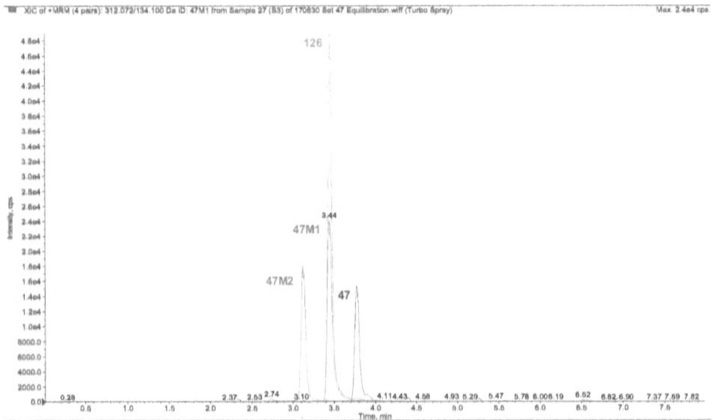

Figure 2.3. Representative chromatogram of the analytes in Set **47**, displaying the parent PDBQ, **47** (R_T = 3.78 min); the major metabolites, **47M1** (R_T = 3.44 min) and **47M2** (R_T = 3.12 min); and the ISTD **126** (R_T = 3.45 min); analysed on the API 2000.

2.3.1.3. Sample preparation

The sample preparation method was developed to extract the PDBQ compounds from murine whole blood. The protein precipitant, which demonstrated the greatest recovery and most consistent extraction at the HQC and LQC concentrations was 0.1% (v/v) NH_4OH in ACN. Ammonium hydroxide was added to the extraction solution to increase the solubility of the analytes in the organic solvent. The extraction solvent was spiked with the ISTD to a final concentration of 300 ng/ml for analysis on the API 2000 and 100 ng/ml for analysis on the API 3200. Double blank samples were extracted with ISTD-free extraction solvent. The sample preparation procedure was performed on ice, when possible. First, calibration curve and experimental study samples were removed from -80°C storage and left to thaw. Samples were then briefly vortexed and 20 µl whole blood aliquots were made. A hundred microliters of ice-cold extraction solvent was added to the whole blood aliquot, the sample was vortexed for 1 min, and then centrifuged at 5590 x *g* for 5 min. The resulting supernatant was added to the analysis plate and then injected onto the HPLC-MS/MS instrument for analyte detection.

The extraction efficiency of the PDBQ parents and metabolites was determined by pooling the analytes within each set. The recovery of the pooled analytes is hypothesised to be consistent to the recovery of the analyte alone as the pooled analytes did not display saturation in the extraction solvent and thus the individual analyte is unlikely to display solvent saturation effects during extraction. Nonetheless, the calibration curves for the quantification of the individual metabolite only were closely monitored at the low and high concentrations to ensure acceptable accuracy and precision.

The absolute recovery of the PDBQ parents and metabolites from murine whole blood, using the protein precipitation method described above, is presented in **Table 2.10**. The difference in the absolute recovery between the HQC and LQC of each analyte was no greater than 15%, which suggests that extraction efficiency is likely to be consistent over the entire calibration range. Additionally, all extractions were within the limits of variability with CV values ≤ 15% except for the LQC where the CV was ≤ 20%.

Table 2.10. Absolute recoveries of the PDBQ parents and metabolites from murine whole blood using protein precipitation with 0.1% (v/v) NH_4OH in ACN

Analyte and QC concentration[a]		Pre-extraction spiked blood[b]			Post-extraction spiked matrix[b]			Mean absolute recovery (%)
		Mean peak area		ISTD-normalised CV (%)	Mean peak area		ISTD-normalised CV (%)	
		Analyte	ISTD		Analyte	ISTD		
49	LQC	2210	122400	19	3620	145400	9	73
	HQC	163000	132000	4	285000	156000	15	68
49M1	LQC	1750	122400	6	2260	145400	10	92
	HQC	163300	132000	5	199200	156000	10	97
49M2	LQC	1520	122400	8	1960	145400	3	92
	HQC	58000	132000	8	76300	156000	9	90
43	LQC	1560	119800	14	1720	112600	18	85
	HQC	73440	102900	9	109100	130200	8	85
43M1	LQC	1690	119800	10	1690	112600	15	94
	HQC	150200	102900	7	213800	130200	10	89
43M2	LQC	1510	119800	18	2040	112600	11	70
	HQC	49900	102900	5	78400	130200	8	81
47	LQC	1580	96100	8	3600	148000	10	68
	HQC	104600	124800	5	127200	109200	5	72
47M1	LQC	1100	96100	12	2340	148000	11	72
	HQC	117200	124800	6	146000	109200	12	70
47M2	LQC	1880	96100	8	3000	148000	9	97
	HQC	62200	124800	7	62100	109200	4	88

[a]LQC = 40 ng/ml and HQC = 3200 ng/ml. [b]n = 3.

2.3.1.4. Selectivity

Figure 2.4 displays a representative chromatogram of double blank murine whole blood. There were no distinct analyte peaks at the expected retention times of **47** (R_T= 3.78 min), **47M1** (R_T= 3.44 min), **47M2** (R_T= 3.12 min), and the ISTD **126** (R_T= 3.45 min). This was similarly observed for all analytes that were analysed on the API 2000 and API 3200. These results indicate minimal interference of endogenous matrix components in the detection of the PDBQ parents and metabolites and acceptable HPLC-MS/MS assay selectivity.

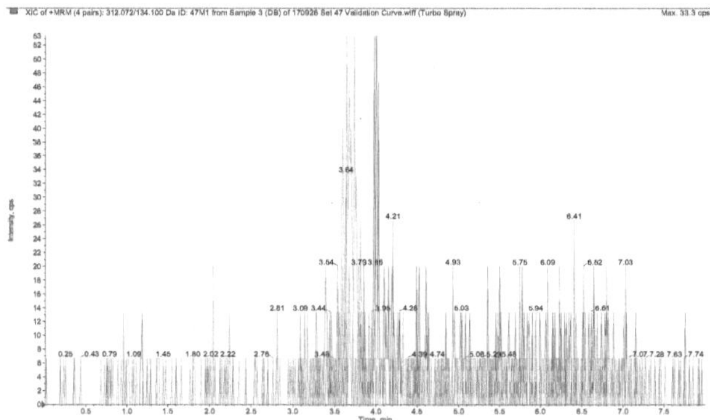

Figure 2.4. Representative chromatogram of double blank murine whole blood. No discernible peaks were detected at the expected retention times of the analytes in Set **47**; analysed on the API 2000.

2.3.1.5. Sensitivity

Figure 2.5 presents a representative chromatogram of the LLOQ of **47M1** (31.3 ng/ml), analysed on the API 2000, which displayed a S/N value of 12.5.

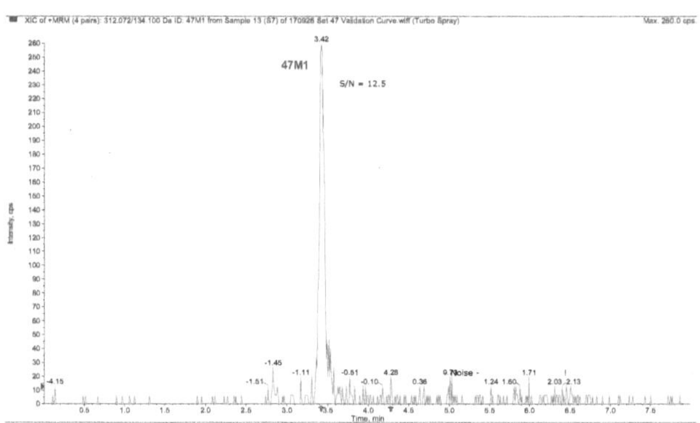

Figure 2.5. Representative chromatogram of the LLOQ of **47M1** (31.3 ng/ml), extracted from murine whole blood; analysed on the API 2000.

All other PDBQ analytes demonstrated similar LLOQ chromatograms, and a summary of their S/N values at the LLOQ is displayed in **Table 2.11**. All analytes displayed LLOQ S/N values ≥ 5. These results suggest that the HPLC-MS/MS assays, developed on the API 2000, are sensitive and are able to reliably detect the analyte in the LLOQ sample.

Table 2.11. LLOQ S/N values obtained from the validation calibration curves of each PDBQ analyte; analysed on the API 2000

Analyte	LLOQ	
	Concentration (ng/ml)	**Mean S/N[a]**
49	15.6	16
49M1	15.6	16
49M2	15.6	12
43	31.3	5
43M1	31.3	6
43M2	31.3	5
47	31.3	7
47M1	31.3	20
47M2	31.3	29

[a]$n = 2$.

Similarly, the assay sensitivity for Set **43** was determined on the API 3200, and a summary of these results is shown in **Table 2.12**. Analyte detection for Set **43** was more sensitive on the API 3200 compared to the API 2000 as displayed by the LLOQ values which were 31.3 and 15.6 ng/ml on the API 2000 and API 3200, respectively. All analytes displayed acceptable S/N values which were between 8–15.

Table 2.12. LLOQ S/N values obtained from the validation calibration curves of each analyte in Set **43**; analysed on the API 3200

Analyte	LLOQ	
	Concentration (ng/ml)	Mean S/N[a]
43	15.6	8
43M1	15.6	15
43M2	15.6	15

[a]$n = 2$.

2.3.1.6. Carryover

A representative blank chromatogram of murine whole blood is presented in **Figure 2.6** and depicts the carryover of **47M1** from the ULOQ (4000 ng/ml) to the blank sample.

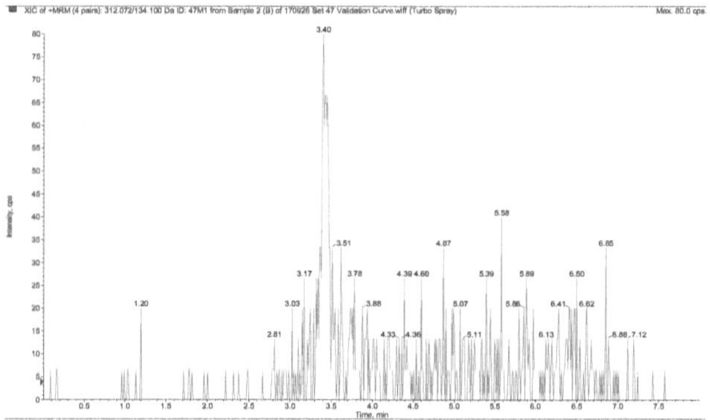

Figure 2.6. Representative chromatogram of blank murine whole blood injected after the ULOQ of **47M1** (4000 ng/ml); analysed on the API 2000.

A summary of the carryover of the PDBQ compounds is presented in **Table 2.13** and **Table 2.14**, and the ISTD carryover is presented in **Table 2.15**. Although the analyte peaks in the blank samples were indistinct, the carryover was still calculated using the analyte peak areas determined by Analyst. The carryover for Set **43** was assessed on both the API 2000 and the API 3200 as each instrument displayed different detection sensitivities and, therefore, the degree of carryover was expected to be different on each instrument. In general, all analytes displayed acceptable carryover from the ULOQ to the blank, which was

≤ 20% of the analyte peak area in the LLOQ. The ISTD also displayed acceptable carryover from the blank to the double blank. These results suggest that the analyte and ISTD carryover will not affect the accuracy and precision of the assay.

Table 2.13. Summary of the carryover of PDBQ parents and metabolites from the ULOQ (4000 ng/ml) to the blank; analysed on the API 2000

Analyte	Mean analyte peak area[a]		Carryover (%)
	Blank	LLOQ[b]	
49	78	1580	5
49M1	84	1890	4
49M2	76	1530	5
43	54	2340	2
43M1	29	1760	2
43M2	25	1100	2
47	45	2120	2
47M1	38	1070	4
47M2	33	1970	2

[a]$n = 2$. [b]LLOQ was 15.6 ng/ml for Set **49** and 31.3 ng/ml for Set **47** and Set **43**.

Table 2.14. Summary of the carryover of the analytes in Set **43** from the ULOQ (4000 ng/ml) to the blank; analysed on the API 3200

Analyte	Mean analyte peak area[a]		Carryover (%)
	Blank	LLOQ[b]	
43	136	2100	6
43M1	167	4280	4
43M2	104	2360	4

[a]$n = 2$. [b]LLOQ was 15.6 ng/ml.

Table 2.15. Summary of the carryover of the ISTD, **126**, from the blank to the double blank; analysed on the API 2000 and API 3200

Instrument	Mean ISTD peak area[a]		Carry over (%)
	Double blank	LLOQ[b]	
API 2000	50	125000	0.4
API 3200	180	280000	0.4

[a]n = 2. [b]ISTD concentration in the LLOQ was 300 and 100 ng/ml for the API 2000 and API 3200, respectively.

2.3.1.7. Calibration curve

Figure 2.7 displays a representative calibration curve of **47M1** obtained during validation. A 1/concentration (1/x) weighted quadratic regression was used to model the relationship between the ISTD-normalised analyte peak area and the analyte concentration. **Table 2.16** and **Table 2.17** display a summary of the regression and the overall accuracy and precision of each analyte's validation calibration curve. In general, all calibration curves were modelled with a 1/x weighted quadratic regression, and all generated curves displayed r values exceeding 0.99. The standards and QCs displayed acceptable accuracy and precision, as discussed in **Section 2.1.3.3** and **Section 2.1.3.4**. The results from the validation calibration curves demonstrate that the developed assays are accurate, precise, and reliable over each analyte's respective analytical range.

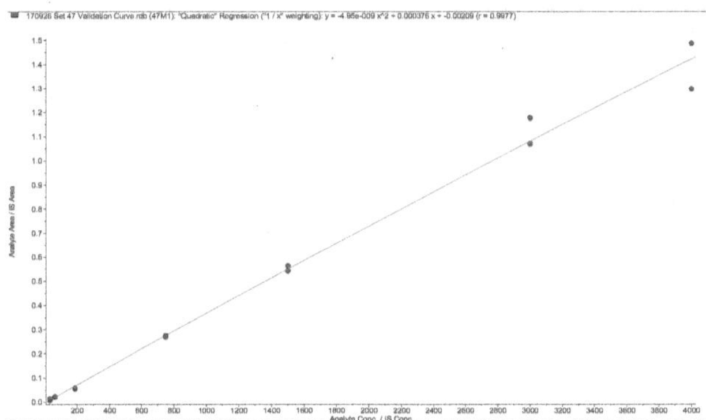

Figure 2.7. Representative calibration curve of **47M1**, using a quadratic regression with a 1/x weighting (r = 0.998), covering the concentration range from 31.3–4000 ng/ml; analysed on the API 2000.

Table 2.16. Summary of the regression and overall accuracy and precision obtained from the validation calibration curves of each PDBQ analyte; analysed on the API 2000

Analyte	Calibration range (ng/ml)	Regression (weighting)	r	Standards[a]		QCs[a]	
				Accuracy range (%)	Precision range (%)	Accuracy range (%)	Precision range (%)
49	15.6–4000	Quadratic (1/x)	0.999	93–115	0.2–8	93–117	1–4
49M1	15.6–4000	Quadratic (1/x)	0.999	86–113	0.8–17	98–110	2–14
49M2	15.6–4000	Quadratic (1/x)	0.998	92–106	0.2–15	105–117	1–11
43	31.3–4000	Quadratic (1/x)	0.998	86–105	4–12	89–117	5–15
43M1	31.3–4000	Quadratic (1/x)	0.998	89–116	0.2–13	97–110	0.7–8
43M2	31.3–4000	Quadratic (1/x)	0.997	98–112	3–17	91–105	9–12
47	31.3–4000	Quadratic (1/x)	0.991	90–107	1–14	98–102	3–16
47M1	31.3–4000	Quadratic (1/x)	0.998	86–111	2–13	99–114	1–5
47M2	31.3–4000	Quadratic (1/x)	0.997	98–113	0.6–11	105–114	0.4–3

[a] $n = 2$.

Table 2.17. Summary of the regression and overall accuracy and precision obtained from the validation calibration curves of each analyte in Set **43**; analysed on the API 3200

Analyte	Calibration range (ng/ml)	Regression (weighting)	r	Standards[a]		QCs[a]	
				Accuracy range (%)	Precision range (%)	Accuracy range (%)	Precision range (%)
43	15.6–4000	Quadratic (1/x)	0.999	85–100	7–13	88–98	5–19
43M1	15.6–4000	Quadratic (1/x)	0.998	88–107	2–15	98–110	4–14
43M2	15.6–4000	Quadratic (1/x)	0.996	88–101	4–18	95–114	6–14

[a] $n = 2$.

2.3.1.8. Matrix effects

A summary of the matrix effects of the PDBQ parents and major metabolites in murine whole blood are presented in **Table 2.18** and **Table 2.19**. The matrix effects for Set **43** were evaluated on both the API 2000 and API 3200 as each instrument has a different API interface and, therefore, the ionisation mechanism of each instrument is presumed to be different. The MF values for all analytes were between 1–1.4 on the API 2000 and between 0.8–0.9 on the API 3200 which suggests ion enhancement on the API 2000 and ion suppression on the API 3200. The inclusion of the ISTD appeared to compensate for the apparent ion enhancement of several analytes, such as that observed for **47M2** on the API 2000, as shown in **Table 2.18**. The ISTD-normalised MF values were generally consistent at each analyte's HQC and LQC concentration which indicates that the matrix effect will not have a significant influence on the accuracy and precision of the assay across the entire calibration range. Although the sample preparation method was not rigorous in removing endogenous matrix components, the procedure, in addition to the gradient HPLC method, was sufficient in limiting any matrix effects.

Table 2.18. Summary of the murine whole blood matrix effects of the PDBQ parents and metabolites; analysed on the API 2000

Analyte and QC concentration[a]		Matrix-free[b]		Post-extraction spiked matrix[b]		MF	ISTD-normalised MF
		Mean analyte peak area	CV (%)	Mean analyte peak area	CV (%)		
126	-[c]	152800	4	189000	4	1.2	-
49	**LQC**	28500	6	36240	2	1.3	1
	HQC	1712000	3	1690000	3	1	0.8
49M1	**LQC**	19440	7	22420	3	1.2	0.9
	HQC	1204000	3	1282500	4	1.1	0.9
49M2	**LQC**	4760	5	6694	4	1.4	1.1
	HQC	414200	11	428200	6	1	0.8
43	**LQC**	1676	15	1720	9	1	0.8
	HQC	164600	11	218320	10	1.3	1.1
43M1	**LQC**	3396	13	3396	6	1	0.8
	HQC	352750	3	407000	4	1.2	0.9
43M2	**LQC**	1240	10	1374	12	1.1	0.9
	HQC	133560	8	156920	7	1.2	0.9
47	**LQC**	2730	10	3644	5	1.3	1.1
	HQC	201600	9	254400	3	1.3	1
47M1	**LQC**	3714	5	4470	5	1.2	1
	HQC	246500	10	273500	4	1.1	0.9
47M2	**LQC**	2090	11	2968	8	1.4	1.1
	HQC	194000	3	248500	7	1.3	1

[a]LQC = 40 ng/ml and HQC = 3200 ng/ml. [b]$4 \leq n \leq 6$. [c] ISTD matrix effects was tested at 300 ng/ml.

Table 2.19. Summary of the murine whole blood matrix effects of Set **43**; analysed on the API 3200

Analyte and QC concentration[a]		Matrix-free[b]		Post-extraction spiked matrix[b]		MF	ISTD-normalised MF
		Mean analyte peak area	CV (%)	Mean analyte peak area	CV (%)		
126	-[c]	435280	2	448800	3	1	-
43	**LQC**	12300	2	11066	6	0.9	0.9
	HQC	479750	4	425600	14	0.9	0.9
43M1	**LQC**	36750	1	32250	7	0.9	0.9
	HQC	1280000	5	1170000	12	0.9	0.9
43M2	**LQC**	16300	9	13100	2	0.8	0.8
	HQC	600500	11	553600	14	0.9	0.9

[a]LQC = 40 ng/ml and HQC = 3200 ng/ml. [b]$4 \leq n \leq 6$. [c]ISTD matrix effects was tested at 100 ng/ml.

2.3.1.9. Stock solution stability

A summary of the stock solution stabilities of the PDBQ parents and metabolites is presented in **Table 2.20**. All analytes displayed acceptable high stability in DMSO for 1 h at ambient temperature as demonstrated by the stability values which were between 93–99%. These results suggest that the DMSO stock solutions need to be used within 1 h of being prepared to allow minimal analyte degradation during calibration standard and QC preparation.

Table 2.20. Summary of the stock solution stabilities of the PDBQ compounds in DMSO for 1 h at ambient temperature

Analyte	Reference			Test condition			Stability (%)
	Mean peak area[a]		ISTD-normalised CV (%)	Mean peak area[a]		ISTD-normalised CV (%)	
	Analyte	ISTD		Analyte	ISTD		
49	155000	57300	6	150200	56700	4	98
49M1	58280	56400	7	59200	58700	3	98
49M2	6718	56900	4	6773	58500	7	98
43	66000	57600	6	62012	56600	5	96
43M1	56419	58000	6	53124	56700	9	96
43M2	23507	58900	8	20917	56700	11	92
47	38740	47900	4	38725	49000	3	98
47M1	47980	47600	7	48933	49100	1	99
47M2	19860	48900	4	19020	47400	5	99

[a]$4 \leq n \leq 6$.

2.3.1.10. Working solution stability

A summary of the working solution stabilities of the PDBQ parents and metabolites is presented in **Table 2.21**. The stability was tested at the concentrations corresponding to WS12 and WS9, which were used to spike the LQC and HQC, respectively, as shown in **Table 2.4**. The stability of the analytes in ACN for 1 h on ice were within the acceptable limit and ranged from 86–99%, which demonstrates high stability under the given test conditions. Additionally, stability was consistent at each analyte's high and low concentration. Therefore, to allow minimal analyte degradation in ACN, the whole blood aliquots need to be spiked with the calibration standard and QC working solutions within 1 h of them being prepared. The working solution stability of the PDBQ compounds was assessed by pooling the analytes within each set, and the determined stability of the pooled analytes are hypothesised to be similar to the stability when the analyte is singly present in the working solution.

Table 2.21. Summary of the working solution stabilities of the PDBQ compounds in ACN for 1 h on ice

Analyte and WS concentration[a]		Reference			Test condition			Stability (%)
		Mean peak area[b]		ISTD-normalised CV (%)	Mean peak area[b]		ISTD-normalised CV (%)	
		Analyte	ISTD		Analyte	ISTD		
49	WS12	4100	105500	6	3780	105700	17	92
	WS9	291500	104000	6	275700	107700	9	91
49M1	WS12	3370	105500	8	2990	105700	1	89
	WS9	333000	104000	7	308300	107700	4	89
49M2	WS12	1510	105500	11	1300	105700	8	86
	WS9	137800	104000	6	127000	107700	11	89
43	WS12	1680	91980	9	1550	88700	4	96
	WS9	167500	88900	5	168500	91400	7	98
43M1	WS12	3390	91980	4	3050	88700	6	93
	WS9	341400	88900	3	338400	91400	19	96
43M2	WS12	1240	91980	12	1170	88700	4	98
	WS9	130000	88900	7	132100	91400	4	99
47	WS12	2730	107000	5	2820	112000	11	99
	WS9	201700	82100	1	200300	82500	4	99
47M1	WS12	3710	107000	5	3550	112000	7	91
	WS9	264400	82100	5	231200	82500	3	87
47M2	WS12	2160	107000	2	2040	112000	5	90
	WS9	194000	82100	3	190200	82500	5	98

[a]WS12 = 1 µg/ml and WS9 = 80 µg/ml, WS12 and WS9 were used to spike the LQC and HQC, respectively. [b]$4 \leq n \leq 6$.

2.3.1.11. Bench-top biological matrix stability

A summary of the stability of the PDBQ parents and metabolites in murine whole blood for 1 h on ice is presented in **Table 2.22**. Analytes were stable in the biological matrix for 1 h on ice with stability values ranging between 87–97%. Additionally, each analyte's stability was consistent at the HQC and LQC concentrations. The whole blood stability was also tested for longer periods on ice, but all analytes exhibited degradation ≥ 25% (data not shown). These results suggest that the calibration standard and QC preparation needs to occur within 1 h of the analyte being spiked into the matrix, and during sample preparation, the analyte needs to be extracted from the matrix within 1 h of the sample being place on ice. Additionally, during experimental PK sampling, samples need to be kept on ice for a maximum of 1 h before being transferred to -80°C for storage.

Table 2.22. A summary of the stability of the PDBQ compounds in murine whole blood for 1 h on ice

Analyte and QC concentration[a]		Reference			Test condition			Stability (%)
		Mean peak area[b]		ISTD-normalised CV (%)	Mean peak area[b]		ISTD-normalised CV (%)	
		Analyte	ISTD		Analyte	ISTD		
49	LQC	2470	122300	14	2400	128400	15	93
	HQC	185800	144600	13	153400	125000	3	96
49M1	LQC	2160	122300	18	2000	128400	13	88
	HQC	104500	144600	8	84000	125000	2	93
49M2	LQC	2220	122300	19	2200	128400	13	94
	HQC	28100	144600	13	23000	125000	4	95
43	LQC	1460	119800	14	1200	113500	20	87
	HQC	73400	102980	9	75600	113600	11	93
43M1	LQC	1700	119800	9	1440	113500	7	89
	HQC	150200	102980	7	150000	113600	8	91
43M2	LQC	1910	119800	14	1580	113500	6	87
	HQC	49800	102980	5	51800	113600	10	94
47	LQC	1580	96160	8	1900	123800	6	93
	HQC	104600	124800	5	92400	114200	8	97
47M1	LQC	1940	96160	7	2240	123800	8	90
	HQC	113500	124800	3	95700	114200	8	92
47M2	LQC	1930	96160	8	2350	123800	6	95
	HQC	60800	124800	9	50220	114200	11	90

[a]LQC = 40 ng/ml and HQC = 3200 ng/ml. [b]$4 \leq n \leq 6$.

2.3.1.12. Post-preparative stability

A summary of the on-instrument stability of the processed PDBQ parents and metabolites from murine whole blood, and the ISTD **126**, is presented in **Table 2.23**. The obtained stability values were within the range of 87–99%, which indicates that all analytes were stable in the extract for 24 h at ambient temperature. In addition, each analyte's stability was consistent at both the high and low concentrations. The post-preparative stability of the ISTD was ≥ 100%; this could most likely be attributed to the day-to-day instrument detection variability, which was not compensated for by an ISTD. Nonetheless, the ISTD does appear to be stable under the given conditions. Together, these results suggest that the extracted samples need to be analysed within 24 h of sample preparation to maintain acceptable assay accuracy and precision.

Table 2.23. Summary of the post-preparative stability of the PDBQ compounds and the ISTD **126** in murine whole blood matrix extract, for 24 h at ambient temperature

Analyte and QC concentration[a]		Reference			Test condition			Stability (%)
		Mean peak area[b]		ISTD-normalised CV (%)	Mean peak area[b]		ISTD-normalised CV (%)	
		Analyte	ISTD		Analyte	ISTD		
49	LQC	2470	122300	14	4400	224000	17	97
	HQC	185800	144600	13	251000	197000	10	99
49M1	LQC	2160	122300	18	3600	224000	20	91
	HQC	104500	144600	8	128100	197000	6	90
49M2	LQC	2220	122300	19	3800	224000	14	93
	HQC	28100	144600	13	37000	197000	7	97
43	LQC	1460	119800	14	1520	129600	19	96
	HQC	73400	102980	9	84540	119600	11	99
43M1	LQC	1700	119800	9	1760	129600	10	96
	HQC	150200	102980	7	163400	119600	4	94
43M2	LQC	1910	119800	14	1800	129600	18	87
	HQC	49800	102980	5	50200	119600	7	87
47	LQC	1580	96160	8	2040	128000	5	97
	HQC	104600	124800	5	93500	117800	5	95

[a]LQC = 40 ng/ml and HQC = 3200 ng/ml. [b]$4 \leq n \leq 6$.

Table 2.23. (Continued)

Analyte and QC concentration[a]		Reference			Test condition			Stability (%)
		Mean peak area[b]		ISTD-normalised CV (%)	Mean peak area[b]		ISTD-normalised CV (%)	
		Analyte	ISTD		Analyte	ISTD		
47M1	LQC	1940	96160	7	2320	128000	7	90
	HQC	113500	124800	3	98400	117800	5	92
47M2	LQC	1930	96160	8	2400	128000	13	93
	HQC	60800	124800	9	55380	117800	5	96
126	-[c]	-	123900	-	-	131800	-	106

[a]LQC = 40 ng/ml and HQC = 3200 ng/ml. [b]$4 \leq n \leq 6$. [c]ISTD stability was tested at 100 ng/ml.

2.3.1.13. Oral formulation stability

The stability of the PDBQ parents and metabolites in the oral dosing vehicle is presented in **Table 2.24**. **47M2** was not included in the oral formulation stability analysis as this compound was excluded from the PK evaluations due to its relatively low *in vitro* antimalarial activity, as shown in **Chapter I, Table 1.1**. All analytes were acceptably stable in 0.5% (w/v) HPMC in H_2O with 0.2% (v/v) Tween80® for 1 h on ice with stability values ranging between 86–98%. These results suggest that the oral dosing formulation needs to be administered within 1 h of preparation to ensure minimal analyte degradation under the given condition.

Table 2.24. Summary of the oral formulation stability of the PDBQ compounds in 0.5% (w/v) HPMC in H_2O with 0.2% (v/v) Tween80® for 1 h on ice

Analyte	Reference			Test condition			Stability (%)
	Mean peak area[a]		ISTD-normalised CV (%)	Mean peak area[a]		ISTD-normalised CV (%)	
	Analyte	ISTD		Analyte	ISTD		
49	628333	177000	4	542667	178333	2	86
49M1	13300	212000	4	9645	169500	9	91
49M2	137500	212000	1	107167	169333	15	98
43	32450	292500	15	30200	309500	9	89
43M1	58550	35000	4	56350	34500	4	98
43M2	32750	301000	11	31400	332000	4	87
47	50350	176500	1	43800	161500	10	96
47M1	23050	169000	14	22850	172000	15	98

[a]*n* = 3.

2.3.1.14. Intravenous formulation stability

The IV formulation stability of the PDBQ parents and metabolites are presented in **Table 2.25**. **47M2** was not included in the IV formulation stability analysis as this compound was excluded from the PK evaluations due to its relatively low *in vitro* antimalarial activity, as shown in **Chapter I, Table 1.1**. All analytes displayed high stability in the IV dosing vehicle, of DMA:PPG:EtOH:PEG400 (5:24:6:15, v/v), for 1 h on ice with stability values ranging from 89–98%. These results suggest that the IV dosing formulation needs to be administered within 1 h of preparation to ensure minimal analyte degradation under the given conditions.

Table 2.25. Summary of the IV formulation stability of the PDBQ compounds in DMA:PPG:EtOH:PEG400 (5:24:6:15, v/v) for 1 h on ice

Analyte	Reference			Test condition			Stability (%)
	Mean peak area[a]		ISTD-normalised CV (%)	Mean peak area[a]		ISTD-normalised CV (%)	
	Analyte	ISTD		Analyte	ISTD		
49	603000	188667	4	512333	176667	11	91
49M1	8562	127800	4	11267	182000	6	93
49M2	136500	186500	3	129000	182000	1	97
43	89250	338500	5	81000	313500	1	98
43M1	65900	327000	14	58950	327000	7	89
43M2	9130	295667	15	8973	294667	7	98
47	119333	162667	11	116000	173667	3	91
47M1	34270	159667	13	34430	174000	2	92

[a]$n = 3$.

2.3.2. Bioanalytical method development and partial validation for the pharmacokinetic studies in malaria-infected mice

The bioanalytical assays used for the PK studies in malaria-infected mice, as presented in **Chapter IV**, is described in this section. HPLC-MS/MS methods were developed for the detection of the lead PDBQ candidates, **43M1** or **47M1**, and the ISTD, **126**, in humanised murine whole blood. The assays were partially validated to address selectivity, sensitivity, extraction efficiency, accuracy, precision, carryover, matrix effects, matrix stability, and post-preparative stability.

The oral dosing range used for these PK studies was between 0.2 – 40 mg/kg; therefore, a relatively wide analytical range was required. Additionally, an MS with greater sensitivity was needed to detect the analyte present in the low dose groups. The expected concentration range of the experimental samples was determined from each analyte's corresponding concentration data that was obtained from the PK studies in healthy mice after a single 20 mg/kg oral administration of each compound, as displayed in **Appendix A**. For the PK studies in malaria-infected mice, the LLOQ was set at one-tenth of the lowest concentration observed in healthy mice which corresponded to the lowest expected concentration of the 0.2 mg/kg dose group. The ULOQ was set at 2 times the highest concentration observed in the healthy mice which corresponded to the highest expected concentration of the 40 mg/kg group. Therefore, the expected PK concentration range for **43M1** was 4–6130 ng/ml and 13–8700 ng/ml for **47M1**.

2.3.2.1. Mass spectrometry

All analytes were monitored at unit resolution in the positive MRM mode. The final MRM method for each analyte is presented in **Table 2.26** and **Table 2.27**. The tables display each analyte's precursor ion to product ion m/z transition and the compound- and source-dependent parameters that were used for their detection on the API 5500.

Table 2.26. Source and gas parameter settings used for the detection of **43M1**, **47M1**, and **126** on the API 5500

MS setting	Value
Ionisation mode	Positive
IonSpray voltage (V)	5500
TEM (°C)	450
GS1 (psi)	50
GS2 (psi)	50
CUR (psi)	40
CAD (psi)	Medium

Table 2.27. Compound-dependent parameter settings used for the detection of **43M1**, **47M1**, and **126** on the API 5500

Analyte	Precursor ion (Da)	Product ion (Da)	Dwell time (msec)	DP (V)	EP (V)	CE (eV)	CXP (V)
43M1	312.0	105.0	150	186	10	35	12
47M1	312.0	134.1	150	116	10	29	16
126	394.1	105.0	150	161	10	33	8

2.3.2.2. Chromatography

A preliminary investigation of analyte carryover was performed during HPLC method development as it was hypothesised that carryover would present a challenge due to the wide calibration range, the basic nature of the analytes, and the increased instrument sensitivity. A representative chromatogram of blank humanised murine whole blood, injected after the ULOQ of **47M1** (10000 ng/ml), is displayed in **Figure 2.8**. The chromatogram does display unacceptably high carryover of **47M1** from the ULOQ to the blank sample.

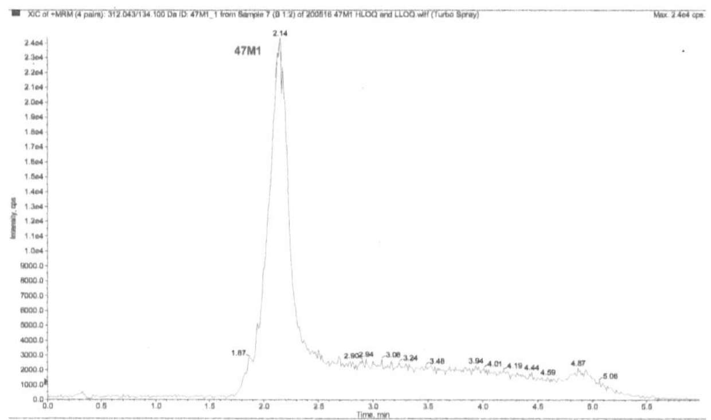

Figure 2.8. Representative chromatogram of blank humanised murine whole blood, depicting the carryover of **47M1** from the ULOQ (10000 ng/ml) to the blank; analysed on the API 5500.

It was determined that carryover was primarily as a result of the analyte being retained on the analytical column, rather than being adsorbed onto the HPLC injection system. Multiple attempts were made to curtail carryover such as; diluting the extracted samples, reducing the column injection volume, and testing different acidic and basic wash solvents. Together these efforts did not significantly reduce the column carryover. Eventually, to resolve the issue, an analytical column wash was performed between each experimental sample injection and additionally, two calibration curves, each with different LLOQ values, were used to cover the entire analytical range.

Chromatography of **43M1** or **47M1** and **126**, was performed with the same HPLC method as outlined here. Separation of M1 and the ISTD was achieved using an Agilent 1260 Infinity II LC System with a Gemini-NX C18 110 Å (50 mm x 2 mm, 5 μM) analytical column. A 400 μl/min gradient run was used, as shown in **Figure 2.9**, using an aqueous mobile phase of H_2O and an organic mobile phase of ACN, both with 0.1% (v/v) NH_4OH (pH 10).

A

Time (min)	Mobile phase (%)	
	Aqueous	Organic
0	70	30
0.3	5	95
3	5	95
3.1	70	30
6	70	30

B

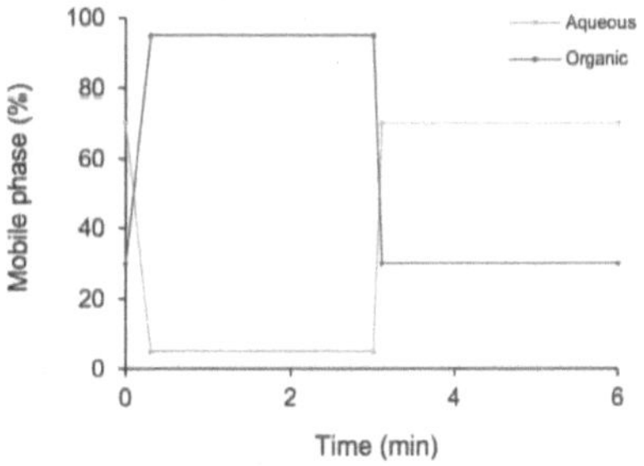

Figure 2.9. A HPLC gradient method and **B** graphical representation of the gradient method used for the separation of **43M1** or **47M1** and the ISTD.

The analytical column temperature was maintained at 30°C. Samples were housed in the autosampler at ambient temperature, and the samples were introduced onto the column with an injection volume of 1 μl. To clean the injection path, a 20 s needle wash, with 0.1% (v/v) NH_4OH in ACN, was performed immediately after the sample was injected onto the column. A representative chromatogram of **47M1** and the ISTD is displayed in **Figure 2.10**.

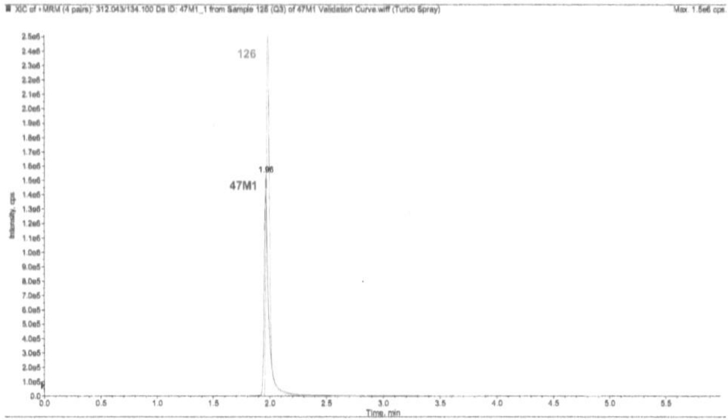

Figure 2.10. Representative chromatogram of **47M1** (R_T= 1.96 min) and the ISTD, **126**, (R_T= 1.98 min); analysed on the API 5500.

The analytical column wash was performed between sample injections and used the same HPLC-MS/MS method as previously described for **43M1** and **47M1**, except for the following modifications. A 15 µl double blank solvent sample, of 2% (v/v) FA and 2% (v/v) DMSO in ACN and H_2O (1:1, v/v), was injected onto the column at the start of the column wash run. During the column equilibration period, an additional series of three washes were performed by injecting 5 µl and 15 µl of 2% (v/v) FA in H_2O onto the needle seat and analytical column, respectively.

A representative chromatogram of the blank solvent column wash, injected after the ULOQ, is shown in **Figure 2.11.A** and depicts the elution of **47M1** during the various wash steps. **Figure 2.11.B** displays a representative chromatogram of blank biological matrix which was injected sequentially after the ULOQ and the blank column wash. The blank biological matrix sample now displays significantly less carryover of **47M1** compared to the blank matrix sample shown in **Figure 2.8**. These results indicate that the blank solvent column wash was effective at removing the strongly-retained analyte from the column. This could most likely be attributed to the strong solubilising activity of DMSO. Additionally, the inclusion of FA most likely encouraged the ionisation of the analyte's basic functional groups which subsequently promoted a greater interaction of the charged analyte to the polar mobile phase compared to the non-polar column.

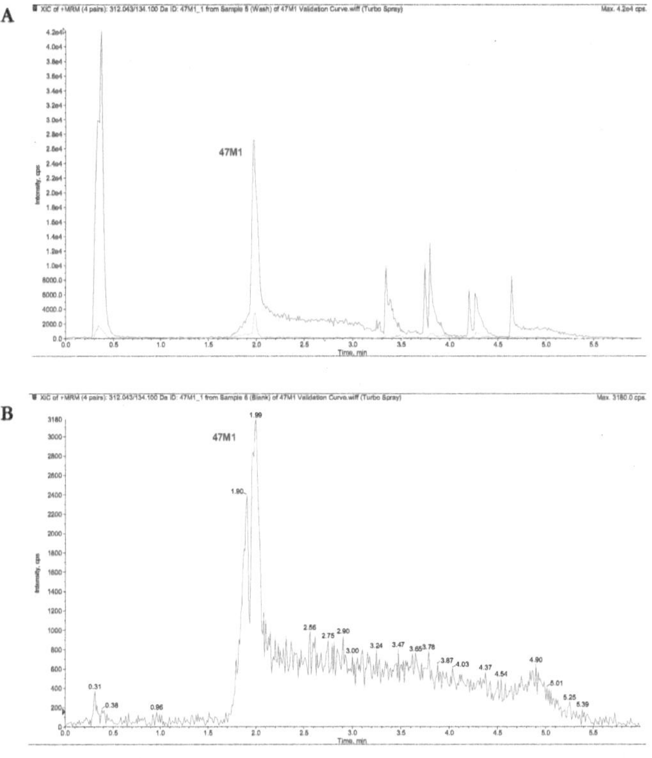

Figure 2.11. Representative chromatograms of **A** blank solvent column wash and **B** blank humanised murine whole blood matrix; illustrating significant carryover of **47M1** from the ULOQ (10000 ng/ml) to the blank solvent and the subsequent analyte carryover from the blank solvent to the blank matrix; analysed on the API 5500.

2.3.2.3. Sample preparation

The sample preparation method for extracting analytes from humanised murine whole blood is as follows, 100 µl ice-cold 0.1% (v/v) NH_4OH in ACN, spiked with the ISTD to a final concentration of 50 ng/ml, was added to 10 µl of the aliquoted blood sample. Double blank matrix samples were processed with ISTD-free extraction solution. The sample was vortexed for 1 min and then centrifuged at 5590 x *g* for 5 min. A twofold dilution of the resulting supernatant was performed in the analysis plate with 0.1% (v/v) NH_4OH in H_2O. The sample was then submitted for HPLC-MS/MS analysis.

The extraction efficiency of **43M1** and **47M1** from humanised murine whole blood is presented in **Table 2.28**. The absolute recovery of **43M1** was 70% and 77% at the LQC and HQC concentration, respectively; and 77% and 76% for **47M1** at the LQC and HQC concentration, respectively. The comparable recoveries at each analyte's LQC and HQC concentration suggest consistent extraction over the entire calibration range.

Table 2.28. Absolute recovery of **43M1** and **47M1** from humanised murine whole blood using protein precipitation with 0.1% (v/v) NH_4OH in ACN

Analyte and QC concentration[a]		Pre-extraction spiked blood			Post-extraction spiked matrix			Absolute recovery (%)
		Mean peak area[b]		ISTD-normalised CV (%)	Mean peak area[b]		ISTD-normalised CV (%)	
		Analyte	ISTD		Analyte	ISTD		
43M1	LQC	52100	1315000	4	61500	1087500	1	70
	HQC	42900000	1150000	3	52825000	1092500	2	77
47M1	LQC	32200	1020000	5	45100	1100000	4	77
	HQC	36000000	1127500	7	45125000	1075000	3	76

[a]LQC = 6 ng/ml and HQC = 9000 ng/ml. [b]n = 4.

2.3.2.4. Selectivity

A representative chromatogram of extracted double blank humanised murine whole blood is displayed in **Figure 2.12**. Relatively indistinct analyte and ISTD peaks were observed at the expected R_T of 1.96 min for **47M1** and 1.98 min for **126**.

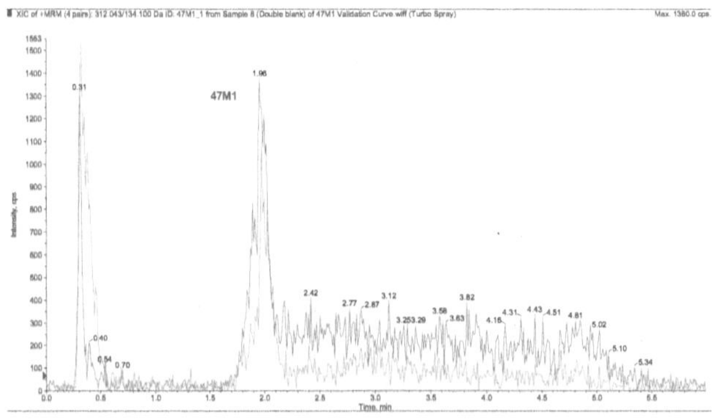

Figure 2.12. Representative chromatogram of double blank humanised murine whole blood; analysed on the API 5500.

As shown in **Table 2.29**, the analyte response of **43M1** and **47M1** in the double blank matrix was ≤ 20% of their respective response in the LLOQ. Additionally, the ISTD response in the double blank matrix was ≤ 5% of the ISTD response in the LLOQ. These results indicate that the developed assays are selective in detecting **43M1, 47M1,** and the ISTD from humanised murine whole blood.

Table 2.29. Summary of the selectivity of the HPLC-MS/MS assays in detecting **43M1**, **47M1**, and the ISTD **126** from humanised murine whole blood; analysed on the API 5500

Analyte	Mean analyte peak area		Selectivity(%)
	Double blank[a]	LLOQ[b,c]	
43M1	2890	23600	12
47M1	3010	33500	9
126	2670	1460000	0.2

[a]n = 4. [b]n = 2. [c]LLOQ is 2 ng/ml for **43M1** and **47M1** and 50 ng/ml for **126**.

2.3.2.5. Sensitivity

A representative chromatogram of the LLOQ of **47M1** is displayed in **Figure 2.13**. As displayed by the S/N value, the analyte response at 2 ng/ml was 46.3 times higher than the background noise.

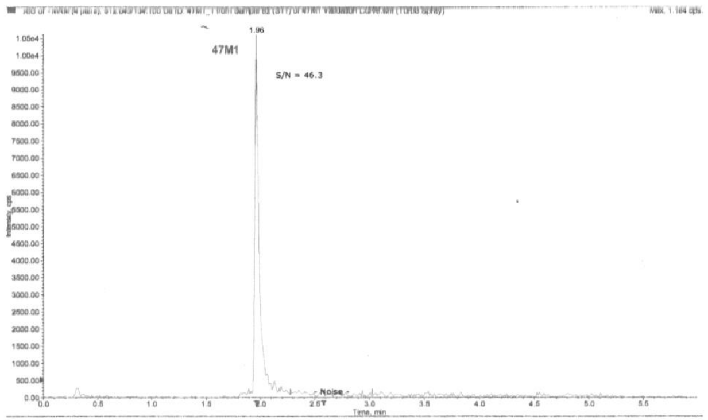

Figure 2.13. Representative chromatogram of the LLOQ of **47M1** (2 ng/ml), extracted from humanised murine whole blood; analysed on the API 5500.

Table 2.30 displays a summary of the assay sensitivity for **43M1** and **47M1**. In general, the S/N values at the LLOQ were above the minimum limit of 5. These results indicate that the developed assays are reliably sensitive in detecting and quantifying **43M1** and **47M1**.

Table 2.30. LLOQ S/N values obtained from the validation calibration curves of **43M1** and **47M1**; analysed on the API 5500

Analyte	**Calibration range (ng/ml)**	**LLOQ**	
		Concentration (ng/ml)	**Mean S/N**[a]
43M1	2–4000	2	20
	75–8000	75	299
47M1	2–4000	2	48
	75–10000	75	250

[a] $n = 2$.

2.3.2.6. Carryover

A summary of the carryover of **43M1**, **47M1**, and the ISTD **126**, is presented in **Table 2.31**. For the higher concentration calibration range, the carryover of **43M1** and **47M1** was below the acceptable limit of 20%. However, for the lower calibration range from 2–4000 ng/ml, the carryover was close to 20%. Although it was within the acceptable limit, it should still be closely monitored during the PK study sample analysis. It was noted that if the percentage carryover exceeded 20%, the LLOQ would need to be increased to the next lowest standard that meets the acceptable carryover criteria to ensure acceptable assay accuracy and precision. The carryover of the ISTD from the blank sample to the double blank sample was within the acceptable limit of 5%.

Table 2.31. Summary of the carryover of **43M1, 47M1**, and the ISTD **126**, obtained from each analyte's validation calibration curve; analysed on the API 5500

Analyte	Calibration range	Mean analyte peak area[a]		Carryover (%)
		Blank[b]	LLOQ	
43M1	2–4000	4250	23600	19
	75–8000	10700	592000	2
47M1	2–4000	6190	33500	18
	75–10000	13800	536000	3
126	-[c]	8240[d]	1460000	0.6

[a]n = 2. [b]Blank sample injected after the ULOQ. [c]ISTD concentration at the LLOQ was 50 ng/ml. [d]ISTD peak area in the double blank sample injected after the blank.

2.3.2.7. Calibration curve

The entire analytical range of **43M1** and **47M1** was covered by two separate calibration curves, each displaying different ULOQ and LLOQ values. Additionally, **47M1** was validated at a higher ULOQ than **43M1** as the expected PK concentrations of **47M1** were presumed to be higher than that of **43M1**, since **47M1** displayed greater systemic absorption in the PK studies in healthy mice compared to **43M1** at the equivalent dose, as discussed in **Chapter III**. **Figure 2.14.A** displays the standard range from 75–10000 ng/ml and **Figure 2.14.B** displays the standard range from 2–4000 ng/ml of **47M1**. The calibration curve covering the range from 75–10000 ng/ml included extra reference standards at the higher concentrations as the instrument response was non-linear.

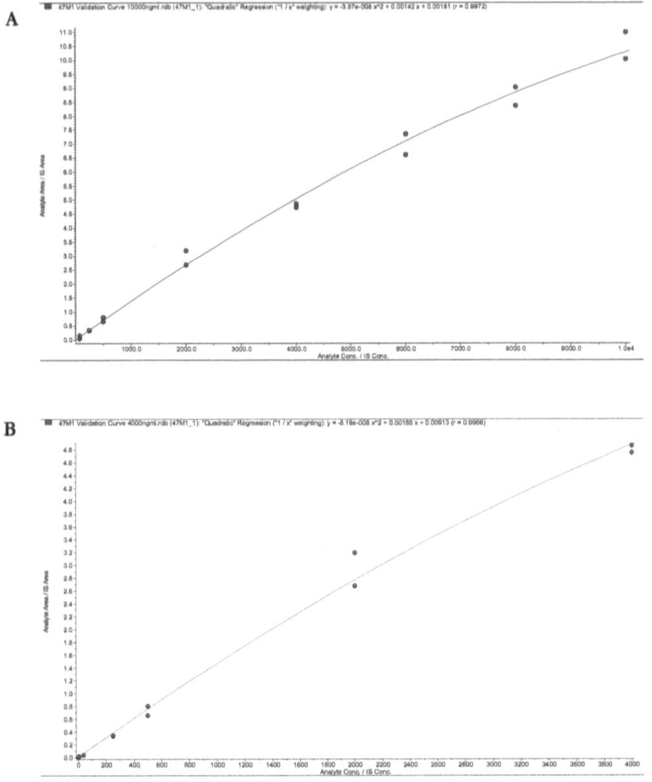

Figure 2.14. Validation calibration curves of **47M1**, covering the concentration ranges from **A** 75–10000 ng/ml, using a 1/x weighted quadratic regression (r = 0.997), and **B** 2–4000 ng/ml, using a 1/x weighted quadratic regression (r = 0.997); analysed on the API 5500.

Table 2.32 displays a summary of the regression and the overall accuracy and precision values that were obtained from the validation calibration curves of **43M1** and **47M1**. In general, all calibration curves were modelled with a quadratic regression with 1/x weighting, and all generated curves displayed r values exceeding 0.99. The standards and QCs displayed acceptable accuracy and precision, as discussed in **Section 2.1.3.3** and **Section 2.1.3.4**. The results from the validation calibration curves demonstrate that the developed assays are accurate, precise, and reliable over each analyte's respective analytical range.

Table 2.32. Summary of the regression and overall accuracy and precision obtained from the validation calibration curves of **43M1** and **47M1**; analysed on the API 5500

Analyte	Calibration range (ng/ml)	Regression (weighting)	r	Standards[a]		QCs[a]	
				Accuracy range (%)	Precision range (%)	Accuracy range (%)	Precision range (%)
43M1	2–4000	Quadratic (1/x)	0.997	96–119	1–20	89–105	4–19
	75–8000	Quadratic (1/x)	0.997	93–106	1–16	99–104	4–14
47M1	2–4000	Quadratic (1/x)	0.997	85–119	1–15	88–103	6–10
	75–10000	Quadratic (1/x)	0.997	94–107	2–19	85–110	3–17

[a] $n = 2$.

2.3.2.8. Matrix effects

The matrix effects of **43M1** and **47M1** in humanised murine whole blood are presented in **Table 2.33**. The observed ISTD-normalised MF values for the analytes were between 1–1.1, which suggests insignificant matrix effects. Furthermore, the matrix effects were consistent at each analyte's high and low concentration. These results demonstrate a minimal influence of matrix effects on the accuracy and precision of the assay across the entire calibration range.

Table 2.33. Summary of the matrix effects of **43M1** and **47M1** extracted from humanised murine whole blood; analysed on the API 5500

Analyte and QC concentration[a]		Matrix-free		Post-extraction spiked matrix		MF	ISTD-normalised MF
		Mean analyte peak area[b]	CV (%)	Mean analyte peak area[b]	CV (%)		
126	-[c]	890000	2	1080000	2	0.8	-
43M1	**LQC**	52100	2	61500	1	0.8	1
	HQC	45050000	11	52825000	10	0.9	1.1
47M1	**LQC**	41400	1	45800	4	0.9	1.1
	HQC	41450000	1	45125000	3	0.9	1.1

[a]LQC = 4 ng/ml and HQC = 7300 ng/ml. [b]n = 4. [c]ISTD matrix effects was tested at 50 ng/ml.

2.3.2.9. Bench-top biological matrix stability

Table 2.34 presents the stability of **43M1** and **47M1** in humanised murine whole blood for 1 h on ice. All analytes displayed acceptable stability, between 90–95%. Additionally, each analyte displayed similar stability at their high and low concentrations. These results demonstrate that the calibration standard, QC, and experimental PK samples should be stored on ice for up to 1 h only before being placed at -80 °C. Additionally, analyte extraction needed to be performed within 1 h of the sample being placed on ice.

Table 2.34. Summary of the stability of **43M1** and **47M1** in humanised murine whole blood for 1 h on ice

Analyte and QC concentration[a]		Reference			Test condition			Stability (%)
		Mean peak area[b]		ISTD-normalised CV (%)	Mean peak area[b]		ISTD-normalised CV (%)	
		Analyte	ISTD		Analyte	ISTD		
43M1	**LQC**	47600	1220000	5	39200	1070000	8	94
	HQC	42900000	1150000	3	48000000	1360000	3	95
47M1	**LQC**	32200	1020000	9	29800	1020000	7	93
	HQC	45300000	1190000	1	37400000	1090000	10	90

[a]LQC = 4 ng/ml and HQC = 7300 ng/ml. [b]n = 3 or 4.

2.3.2.10. Post-preparative stability

Table 2.35 presents the on-instrument stability of **43M1**, **47M1**, and **126** in humanised murine whole blood extract for 24 h at ambient temperature. Both analytes and the ISTD displayed high stability at the HQC and LQC concentrations, between 90–98%. These results indicate that the extracted samples need to be analysed within 24 h of being prepared to ensure acceptable assay accuracy and precision.

Table 2.35. Summary of the post-preparative stability of **43M1**, **47M1**, and the ISTD **126**, extracted from humanised murine whole blood, for 24 h at ambient temperature

Analyte and QC concentration[a]		Reference			Test condition			Stability (%)
		Mean peak area[b]		ISTD-normalised CV (%)	Mean peak area[b]		ISTD-normalised CV (%)	
		Analyte	ISTD		Analyte	ISTD		
43M1	LQC	47600	1220000	5	45700	1210000	7	97
	HQC	42900000	1150000	3	42800000	1170000	2	98
47M1	LQC	32200	1020000	9	29000	1020000	8	90
	HQC	45300000	1190000	1	44000000	1210000	3	96
126	–[c]	–	1180000	–	–	1150000	–	97

[a]LQC = 4 ng/ml and HQC = 7300 ng/ml. [b]n = 3 or 4. [c]ISTD stability was tested at 50 ng/ml.

2.4. CONCLUSION

Several HPLC-MS/MS methods were developed and partially validated for the quantitative analysis of the PDBQ compounds in whole blood. For the PK studies in healthy mice, as presented in **Chapter III**, the HPLC-MS/MS methods were developed to simultaneously quantify the parent, M1, M2, and the ISTD of each *ortho-*, *meta-*, and *para-* set of PDBQ compounds. For the PK studies in malaria-infected mice, as presented in **Chapter IV**, the HPLC-MS/MS methods were developed to quantify **43M1** or **47M1** and the ISTD. All assays demonstrated selectivity, sensitivity, accuracy, and precision over their respective calibration ranges. In addition, all analytes exhibited acceptable stability under the given time and environmental conditions, and therefore, all bioanalytical methodologies for the PK studies were performed without deviation from the tested conditions. Subsequently, the methods were specifically applied to reliably quantify the unknown analyte concentrations in the experimental PK study samples.

CHAPTER III

IN VIVO PHARMACOKINETICS IN A HEALTHY MURINE MODEL

3.1. INTRODUCTION

3.1.1. Chapter aim

This chapter investigates the *in vivo* PK of the PDBQ parent compounds and their major active metabolites, M1 and M2, in a healthy murine model to subsequently allow for the rational selection of lead compounds to be assessed for their *in vivo* antimalarial efficacy in the *P. falciparum* humanised murine model. The PDBQ compounds were developed for oral administration as this route is generally the most practical and convenient[118].

3.1.2. Absorption, distribution, metabolism, and excretion

PK examines the movement of a drug through the body and describes ADME, whereas pharmacodynamics (PD) studies the physiological effect of a drug on the body. Generally, a relationship exists between the pharmacokinetics and pharmacodynamics (PK/PD) where the efficacy of a drug, its PD, is related to the concentration of the drug, its PK, at the target site. Furthermore, an implicit assumption of PK/PD is that the greater the concentration at the site of action, the greater the intensity of the pharmacological effect[118]. Within the scope of preclinical drug discovery, it is important to establish the *in vivo* PK of lead compounds as this will provide insights into whether it has potential to attain concentrations within its therapeutic window for a sufficient amount of time and thus, will provide an understanding of its capability to produce the desired effect. In addition, the safety of the compound can be addressed by assessing whether the concentration attains levels that could be potentially toxic.

In vitro ADME systems are used to aid in the prediction of *in vivo* PK drug behaviours as well as to identify which ADME properties might negatively influence *in vivo* drug levels. These high-throughput ADME screens are beneficial in early drug development as they guide the selection process of lead candidates from a chemical library, where compounds which display poor drug-like properties are deprioritised or withdrawn from further investigation. Furthermore, before proceeding with intensive studies in animal models, it is crucial to discern and address possible ADME liabilities which could limit efficacy[119,120].

The absorption of a drug defines its movement from the site of administration into the bloodstream. Drugs which display poor absorption might demonstrate inadequate efficacy if they are unable to reach concentrations high enough to exert a sufficient therapeutic effect. Intravenously administered drugs are introduced directly into systemic circulation, whereas those which are orally administered undergo gastrointestinal absorption, membrane permeation, and biotransformation before reaching systemic circulation, all of which can diminish exposure[121]. Additionally, orally administered drugs encounter varying pH conditions, first the gastric fluid in the stomach of pH 1.0–2.5 and then the intestinal fluid in the small intestine of pH 6.6[122]. The degree of drug dissolution in the gastrointestinal tract (GIT) is often governed by the surrounding pH environment, which can cause drug precipitation and subsequently limit permeation across the GIT membrane, and thus, reduce oral absorption[80]. A preliminary assessment of the extent of GIT absorption of a compound can be determined through an *in vitro* characterisation of its kinetic solubility and passive permeability at physiologically relevant pH conditions[123].

Solubility and permeability are dependent on the structural and physicochemical properties of a compound such as molecular weight, lipophilicity, and the pK_a[80]. Moreover, the extent of drug absorption is largely dependent on the pK_a of a molecule which influences its ionisation state in the surrounding pH environment. For example, ionised molecules display higher aqueous solubility than neutral molecules due to their more polar nature and unionised molecules are more membrane-permeable than ionised molecules due to their non-polar interactions with phospholipid membranes[124,125]. In general, weakly basic drugs are ionised in an acidic environment which augments their dissolution in gastric fluid. As the drug moves through the small intestine, the pH increases, and the drug tends towards an unionised state. In such cases, the overall solubility is likely to decrease however, the neutral state of the molecule is predicted to increase membrane permeability and therefore promote GIT absorption[126,127].

After absorption in the GIT, the drug passages to the liver via portal circulation. In the liver, the drug undergoes biotransformation to make the molecule more hydrophilic to facilitate excretion via bile or urine. These enzymatic conversions also occur at other sites such as the GIT wall, lungs, and kidneys; however, the liver is the predominant site for metabolism[128]. Metabolism is primarily mediated by the cytochrome P450 (CYP) isoforms;

amongst other enzyme families such as esterases, transferases, and oxidases. These enzymatic modifications are divided into Phase I and Phase II metabolic pathways. Phase I reactions involve oxidation, reduction, and hydrolysis and Phase II reactions involve the conjugation of highly polar groups to the molecule through glucuronidation, sulfation, N-acetylation, and methylation, to name a few[129]. Hepatic metabolism is referred to as the first-pass effect and occurs before the drug reaches systemic circulation. This process ultimately reduces the bioavailability of the orally administered drug through the loss of the parent by the formation of active or inactive metabolites[128]. Therefore, in addition to drug solubility and permeability, exposure is further limited by the extent of first-pass metabolism.

Once the drug has been processed by the liver, it enters into systemic circulation and distributes throughout the body. The degree of distribution is influenced by the lipophilicity of the drug, which determines its permeability towards tissue membranes and its affinity to bind to plasma proteins. Plasma protein binding (PPB) refers to the extent of a drug binding reversibly to blood proteins such as albumin, alpha-1-glycoprotein, lipoproteins, and the globulins[130]. Only unbound drug is able to exert a pharmacological effect, passively diffuse through biological membranes, and be available for excretion processes; therefore, PPB has an impact on a drugs' efficacy, extravascular distribution, and elimination, respectively. Although PPB is an important ADME consideration, it is more valuable to use *in vitro* PPB data retrospectively in the context of *in vivo* PK as it provides insight into the impact of PPB on drug distribution and elimination[131].

The final ADME process is elimination, where the drug and formed metabolites are irreversibly excreted from the body. As previously discussed, the elimination of a drug is dependent on its susceptibility to metabolism and its PPB, both of which are, for the most part, largely influenced by the drugs' lipophilicity[118].

In vitro ADME is indicative of an *in vivo* setting and is useful in predicting *in vivo* drug behaviour, however, *in vitro* ADME models do not always translate to what is observed in a complex, multifactorial *in vivo* ADME setting which simultaneously combines all the effects of solubility, permeability, lipophilicity, metabolic stability, and PPB. Nonetheless, it is still valuable to explore *in vitro* ADME as it facilitates lead compound selection and can further contribute to understanding and interpreting *in vivo* outcomes.

3.1.3. Absorption, distribution, metabolism, and excretion of the parent pyridodibemequines and major metabolites

An *in vitro* ADME screen of the PDBQ parent compounds and their major active metabolites, M1 and M2, was undertaken to characterise their solubility, permeability, lipophilicity, and metabolic stability and, moreover, to determine whether the metabolites display improved drug-like properties in comparison to their parents[75,77].

The PDBQ parent compounds and metabolites have basic amino functional groups, therefore, in an acidic environment, the molecule is expected to become ionised, and in its charged state, the compound should display enhanced solubility in the acidic stomach and in the weakly acidic regions of the GIT. As the basic compound moves through the GIT and encounters more basic pH conditions, it becomes unionised, which could reduce dissolution but promote passive membrane permeation. For optimal GIT absorption, a weakly basic drug should dissolve in gastric fluid and remain in solution in the intestinal fluid to allow membrane diffusion. The *in vitro* kinetic solubility, passive permeability, and lipophilicity of the PDBQ parents and metabolites were investigated and are presented in **Table 3.1**. Kinetic solubility was evaluated by means of an assay which determined the concentration of a 200 μM DMSO drug stock solution in an organic solvent relative to its dissolution in an aqueous biorelevant medium at pH 6.5. A maximum concentration of 200 μM indicates total compound solubility without precipitation at pH 6.5. The parents and metabolites exhibited moderate (**49M1**, **49M2**, **43**, and **43M2**) to high (**49**, **43M1**, **47**, **47M1**, and **47M2**) aqueous solubility at pH 6.5, which, therefore, can facilitate favourable oral absorption in the GIT[75,77]. **43M1** and **47M1** exhibited the highest maximum solubility compared to the other PDBQ compounds. The parallel artificial membrane permeability assay, or PAMPA, was used to determine the passive, transcellular permeability of a compound across a hexadecane liquid layer at pH 6.5, and measured the apparent permeability of unionized compound ($\log P_{app}$)[132,133]. The PDBQ parents and metabolites displayed moderate (**43M2** and **47M2**) to high membrane permeability (**49**, **43**, **47**, **49M1**, **49M2**, **43M1**, and **47M1**), which predicts efficient passive diffusion through the GIT membrane and can translate to high absorption[75,77]. The *in vitro* assay used to determine lipophilicity evaluated the tendency of a molecule to partition between two immiscible polar (aqueous buffer) and non-polar (1-octanol) liquid phases at a given pH; and measured the distribution coefficient ($LogD_{7.4}$) of ionized and neutral molecules at pH 7.4. All metabolites displayed a decrease in lipophilicity, with $LogD_{7.4}$ values ranging between 0.69–0.95, compared to the parents, which displayed $LogD_{7.4}$ values between 2.47–3.79[75,77]. Highly lipophilic compounds are more susceptible to metabolism as they need to be converted to a more polar molecule to facilitate excretion; therefore, the metabolites are expected to display greater metabolic stability as they are less lipophilic than the parent compounds[128]. Additionally, the reduced lipophilicity of the metabolites, as compared to the parents, is hypothesised to result in reduced systemic accumulation and hERG channel inhibition, which could potentially lower the toxicity risk associated with the PDBQ parent compounds[76,80].

Table 3.1. *In vitro* kinetic solubility, passive permeability, and lipophilicity of the PDBQ parents and major metabolites[75,77]

Compound	Kinetic solubility	Permeability	Lipophilicity
	pH 6.5 (μM)	$LogP_{app}$ pH 6.5 (cm/s)	$LogD_{7.4}$
49	164.7	-4.56	3.79
49M1	90.0	-5.20	0.95
49M2	125.0	-4.30	0.85
43	59.8	-4.10	2.47
43M1	200.0	-5.00	0.95
43M2	122.3	-5.90	0.84
47	196.6	-4.56	2.85
47M1	200.0	-4.00	0.69
47M2	165.0	-7.00	0.69

The *in vitro* model developed to assess metabolic stability is based upon the liver, which is the major metabolising organ. This assay makes use of microsomes, a subcellular fraction of the liver, which contains the major metabolising membrane-bound CYP enzymes, amongst other Phase I enzymes and primary conjugation enzymes[134]. The *in vitro* rate of hepatic metabolism of the PDBQ parents and metabolites were previously determined in mouse liver microsomal preparations using a microsomal turnover assay, which determined the percentage of incubated compound that remained after 30 min. This assay was also able to predict the half-life of a compound and the *in vitro* intrinsic clearance (Cl_{int}) by measuring compound depletion over time. This provided an index of the hepatic elimination process and measured the ability of the liver to remove the compound in the absence of plasma proteins[135]. As shown in **Table 3.2**, the parents displayed a greater propensity for hepatic metabolism compared to the metabolites; this could be attributed to the highly lipophilic nature of the parent compounds. The PDBQ parents were extensively metabolised to produce M1 and M2 through N-dealkylation on the tertiary amine, a Phase I reaction mediated by CYP enzymes[75,77,129]. As expected, the metabolites were significantly more stable compared to their metabolically labile parents, except for **43M1**, which displayed a relatively short projected half-life. In general, the metabolic stability of the metabolites is predicted to reduce the first-pass effect, which could, therefore, reflect in improved oral absorption compared to the parent compounds. The *in vitro* Cl_{int} of the parents and **43M1** was high which is generally unfavourable as they are anticipated to be rapidly eliminated from the body, which could contribute to reduced systemic concentrations and a short duration of action. All other metabolites displayed moderate *in vitro* Cl_{int}, which could promote a sustained *in vivo* exposure. It should be noted that all compounds could be further susceptible to metabolism by enzymes not present in the mouse liver microsomal preparations such as other Phase II conjugation enzymes.

Table 3.2. *In vitro* metabolic stability of the PDBQ parents and metabolites in mouse liver microsomes[75,77]

Compound	% remaining after 30 min	Projected microsomal half-life (min)	Cl_{int} (ml/min/kg)
49	2.3	5.5	1224
49M1	97.0	> 100	10
49M2	98.5	> 100	5
43	3.0	5.9	1139
43M1	19.0	12.5	545
43M2	99.9	> 150	–[a]
47	2.1	5.4	1250
47M1	90.4	> 100	33
47M2	91.5	> 100	60

[a]Data not available.

In summary, the *in vitro* ADME profile of the PDBQ metabolites exhibited markedly improved ADME properties in terms of metabolic stability, reduced lipophilicity, and high solubility and permeability compared to the parents. The Biopharmaceutics Drug Classification System is widely utilised in drug discovery and correlates *in vitro* kinetic solubility and passive permeability with *in vivo* oral absorption[123]. Based on this classification scheme, the metabolites are predicted to undergo good intestinal absorption due to their high solubility and permeability. Additionally, the high metabolic stability of the metabolites suggests favourable oral absorption. The encouraging drug-like properties of the metabolites supported a further investigation into their *in vivo* PK in a healthy murine model.

3.1.4. A review of non-compartmental analysis

The PK of a drug describes its quantitative movement through the body after administration and represents its ADME. As previously discussed, it is important to establish the PK of a lead compound as, generally, its concentration has a significant effect on its efficacy and safety, where the concentration, at the site of action, should be within the therapeutic window to exert the desired pharmacological effect; but below the toxicity level in order to prevent adverse drug reactions[118]. Once sufficient, promising *in vitro* characterisation of a lead compound has been demonstrated it can progress to *in vivo* animal studies to determine the PK/PD. PK exhibits a time course of drug concentration from which several PK parameters can be determined through compartmental or non-compartmental analysis (NCA). Compartmental analysis makes use of modelling the PK data upon a number of distinct body compartments, whereas NCA does not require any specific compartment model for the body[136]. Generally, the approach taken for initial exposure characterisation is NCA, which is model-independent, and the PK parameters can be derived directly from the concentration-time data. For the purposes of this comparative study, NCA was adopted to determine the PK parameters, specifically the maximum concentration of the drug (C_{max}), the time taken to reach the maximum concentration (T_{max}), the elimination half-life ($T_{1/2}$), the apparent volume of distribution (V_d), the systemic clearance (Cl), the area under the concentration-time curve extrapolated from zero to infinity ($AUC_{0-\infty}$), and the oral bioavailability (F).

C_{max} and T_{max} values describe the absorption characteristics of a drug and are derived after oral administration[137]. C_{max} provides information on the extent of oral drug absorption, permeability, and first-pass metabolism and T_{max} describes the rate at which absorption into systemic circulation occurs[138,139]. These values are closely dependent on the frequency of experimental sampling and are, therefore, estimations. Nonetheless, they are still valuable in assessing the onset of action. A relatively high C_{max} indicates good oral absorption into systemic circulation, and a relatively low T_{max} value indicates rapid systemic absorption. After C_{max} is reached, a progressive decline in the concentration is observed due to distribution and elimination processes.

$T_{1/2}$ is the time taken for the drug concentration to reduce by one half from a reference concentration during the elimination phase. After IV administration, $T_{1/2}$ is determined by the distribution and elimination of a drug, whereas after oral administration, $T_{1/2}$ is determined not only by distribution and elimination but also by absorption. The $T_{1/2}$ provides information on the period of drug exposure during the terminal phase and can assist in assessing the duration of activity. The $T_{1/2}$ can also provide an indication of possible toxicity issues that can arise from accumulation, which can be represented by a relatively long $T_{1/2}$[137]. The calculated experimental $T_{1/2}$ is largely dependent on the sensitivity of the bioanalytical assay[121].

V_d is a theoretical concept determined after IV administration, and provides information on the apparent distribution of a drug within the body, specifically if it is distributed within tissues or if it is in systemic circulation[118]. Drugs with a relatively high V_d disseminate to extravascular sites where higher levels of drug are found dispersed in the tissue compared to the blood. Drugs with a relatively low V_d are predominantly confined to the vascular system. V_d is largely dependent on the physicochemical properties of a drug such as lipophilicity, which determines whether a drug will readily cross tissue membranes. Additionally, PPB has a large effect on V_d where drugs that are highly protein-bound are mostly distributed within the blood and will, therefore, exhibit a relatively small V_d[118,121,140].

Cl is defined as the volume of blood cleared of drug per unit time and measures the efficiency at which a drug is irreversibly removed from systemic circulation after IV administration. Systemic Cl reflects the cumulative Cl from all eliminating organs and is dependent on factors such as blood flow and PPB[137,141]. A relatively high Cl is associated with a fast elimination process which can reduce the extent of drug exposure and the duration of activity[139].

$AUC_{0-\infty}$ describes the overall extent of drug exposure. Besides the degree of oral absorption, $AUC_{0-\infty}$ is also affected by the elimination process where clearance has an inverse correlation with exposure. V_d does not exhibit a direct relationship with $AUC_{0-\infty}$[121,141]. A relatively high $AUC_{0-\infty}$ reflects high drug exposure.

The F of a drug is the fraction of orally administered drug that reaches systemic circulation. F is a dose-normalised percentage value which compares oral exposure to IV exposure, the latter of which is assumed to exhibit complete absorption. A low F can be attributed to either incomplete intestinal absorption, first-pass metabolism, or a combination of both[118].

It is important to investigate the *in vivo* PK as it provides a comprehensive illustration of the overall drug absorption and disposition, taking into account all the *in vitro* ADME properties simultaneously. *In vivo* PK lends to a more accurate inference of the ability of a compound to reach and maintain efficacious levels, while still remaining below the toxicity boundary.

3.1.5. Determinants for compound progression

Lead compounds that were selected for the antimalarial efficacy evaluation in the *P. falciparum*-infected humanised murine model were chosen based upon their *in vitro* potencies in CQS and CQR strains of *P. falciparum*, specifically their activity against the multidrug sensitive strain *Pf*3D7, which was used for the infection in the humanised murine model, their toxicity in a mammalian cell line, their selectivity against *P. falciparum*, and their *in vivo* PK in healthy mice. The PK requirements for driving efficacy are C_{max}, $AUC_{0-\infty}$, and the time in which the circulating antimalarial concentration remains above its *in vitro* IC_{50}, which gives a measure of the duration of active exposure[142,143,144]. Consequently, these PK criteria were implemented when selecting lead candidates from the PDBQ series of parents and major metabolites. Compounds which displayed relatively high oral exposures and sustained durations of action were selected for progression as these identified PK properties strengthen the likelihood that the compound will reach and maintain therapeutically-effective levels.

3.1.6. Pharmacokinetic study design in healthy mice

The PK studies for the active PDBQ metabolites were designed to compare the PK profiles of the preformed metabolites to the PK profile of the metabolites when administered as the parent; and, furthermore, to assess any *in vivo* PK liabilities of this series. This comparative analysis assisted in determining which compounds, whether it be the parent or preformed metabolite, exhibited the most favourable PK profiles based upon the criteria discussed in **Section 3.1.5** and, thus, which are most likely to produce the highest *in vivo* antimalarial activity in a *P. falciparum*-infected murine model.

The approach to compound administration involved a single-dose administration of the parent PDBQ and subsequent quantification of the parent and formation of the major metabolites, and then separately administering and quantifying each preformed metabolite with the same dosing regimen as the parent, as shown in **Figure 3.1**. After the administration of either preformed M1 or M2, the respective secondary formation of either M2 or M1 was not monitored as trace amounts of the other metabolite was detected in the synthesised sample. Oral administration of the parent PDBQ compound provided an opportunity to assess the contribution of M1 and M2 to the overall cumulative exposure of the quinoline antimalarial pharmacophore, which is inherent in the structure of both the parent and metabolites. **47M2** was excluded from further development and was not evaluated in the *in vivo* PK study as its relatively low antimalarial activity and selectively, as shown in **Chapter I, Table 1.1**, were identified as risk factors for toxicity.

A *Ortho*-substituted PDBQ parent and major metabolites

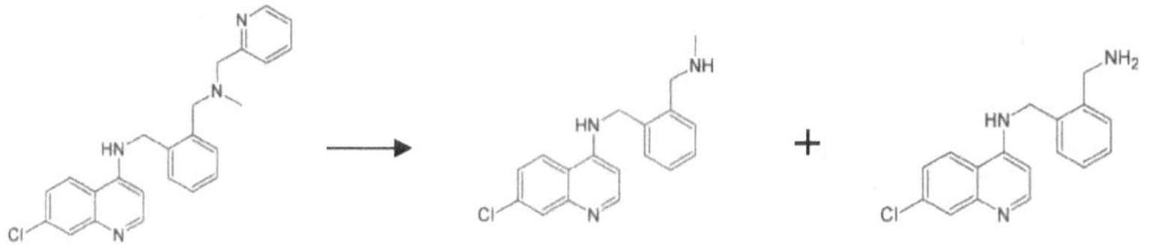

49
PK Experiment 1
Oral: 20 mg/kg
IV: 5 mg/kg

49M1
PK Experiment 2
Oral: 20 mg/kg
IV: 5 mg/kg

49M2
PK Experiment 3
Oral: 20 mg/kg
IV: 5 mg/kg

B *Meta*-substituted PDBQ parent and major metabolites

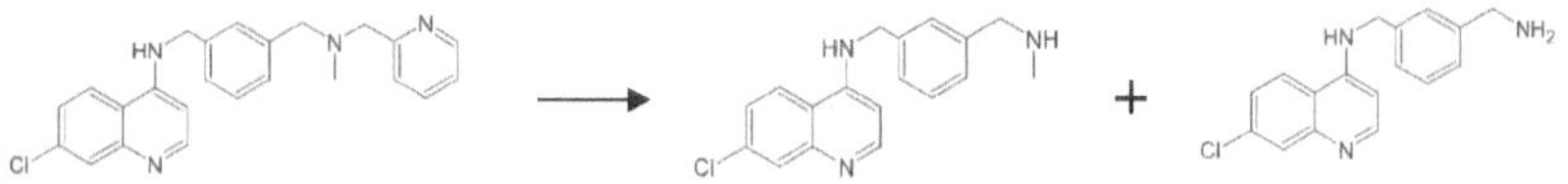

43
PK Experiment 4
Oral: 20 mg/kg
IV: 5 mg/kg

43M1
PK Experiment 5
Oral: 20 mg/kg
IV: 5 mg/kg

43M2
PK Experiment 6
Oral: 20 mg/kg
IV: 5 mg/kg

C *Para*-substituted PDBQ parent and major metabolites

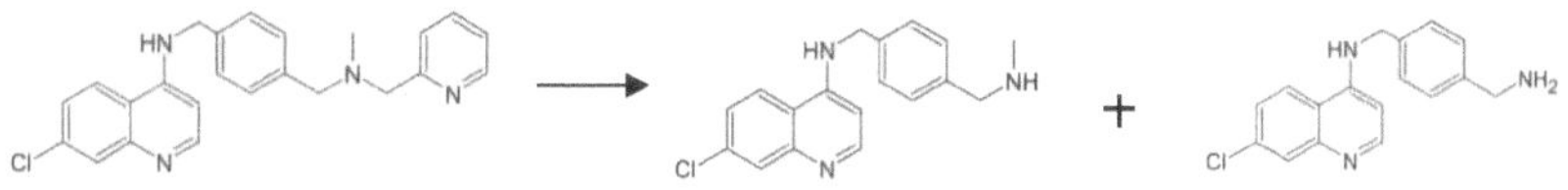

47
PK Experiment 7
Oral: 20 mg/kg
IV: 5 mg/kg

47M1
PK Experiment 8
Oral: 20 mg/kg
IV: 5 mg/kg

47M2
Preformed **47M2** was not administered due to its relatively low *in vitro* activity against *P. falciparum*.

Figure 3.1. Dosing overview of the independent PK experiments performed in healthy mice of **A** the *ortho*-substituted PDBQ parent **49** and its preformed metabolites **49M1** and **49M2, B** the *meta*-substituted PDBQ parent **43** and its preformed metabolites **43M1** and **43M2**, and **C** the *para*-substituted PDBQ parent **47** and its preformed metabolite **47M1**.

3.2. METHODS

3.2.1. Ethics statement

The *in vivo* PK experiments in C57BL/6 mice were performed at the animal unit in the Division of Clinical Pharmacology, UCT. Before commencement of this study, ethical approval was granted by the Animal Ethics Committee of the FHS, UCT. The ethics reference numbers are 013/028 and 017/026.

3.2.2. Animal housing

The PK experiments were performed in healthy 12–16 week old, male C57BL/6 mice, weighing an average of 25 g. Mice were obtained from the Research Animal Facility, UCT and acclimatized to the controlled experimental environment for at least four days prior to the start of the experiment. Mice were supplied with food and water *ad libitum* before and during the experiment. They were monitored daily for signs of distress and discomfort. Animal husbandry and experimental procedures were followed in accordance with the guidelines of the Animal Ethics Committee of UCT.

3.2.3. Materials and instrumentation

The PDBQ parent and metabolite compounds were synthesised at the Department of Chemistry, UCT. The HPLC purity of the compounds is presented in **Chapter II, Table 2.1**. The materials used to formulate the oral and IV dosing vehicles are listed in **Chapter II, Section 2.2.1**. The materials and instrumentation used for the HPLC-MS/MS analyte quantification, as described in **Section 3.2.5**, is presented in **Chapter II, Section 2.2.1** and **Section 2.2.2**.

3.2.4. Compound administration and sampling

All compounds were administered within 1 h of them being prepared in their respective dosing vehicle. Additionally, all dosing solutions were vortexed and sonicated to enhance solubility and the formation of a homogenous suspension. Orally administered compounds were formulated in 0.5% (w/v) HPMC in H_2O with 0.2% (v/v) Tween80®. A single dose of 20 mg/kg of the test compound suspended in the oral solution was administered to each mouse through oral gavage, n = 2 or 3. Compounds administered through an IV bolus injection were dissolved in a solution of DMA, PPG, EtOH, and PEG400 (5:24:6:15, v/v), which was used to enhance drug solubility. Following anaesthesia of mice, a single dose of 5 mg/kg of the test compound dissolved in the IV dosing formulation was administered via the dorsal penile vein, $n = 2$ or 3. The administered drug volume was determined according to the mouse body weight and did not exceed 200 µl and 50 µl for the oral and IV groups, respectively.

The whole blood sample collection time points were set in order to observe the early distribution. For the IV group, the first sample was taken shortly after administration at 0.17 h and again at 0.5 h; and for the oral group, the first sample was collected slightly later, at 0.5 h, to account for the delay before reaching systemic circulation due to oral absorption. For technical reasons, the last sample was taken at either 24, 32, or 48 h after administration. These experimental samples were taken to capture the elimination phase and allow for a reliable estimation of the $T_{1/2}$. Whole blood samples were collected at the predetermined time points post-administration by tail vein bleeding into lithium heparin tubes. Samples were temporarily stored on ice and then transferred to -80°C for storage until HPLC-MS/MS analysis. The cumulative blood volume collected throughout the experimental sampling was < 10% of the total blood volume of the mouse, corrected for body weight, where approximately 20 µl of whole blood was collected at each time point.

3.2.5. Analyte quantification

The parent PDBQ and metabolites were quantified from mouse whole blood samples using the relevant HPLC-MS/MS bioanalytical method as described in **Chapter II, Section 2.3.1**. The PK samples for each analyte's oral and IV group were independently extracted, each with a new set of calibration standard and QC samples, which were analysed in triplicate. In summary, -80°C PK experimental samples, calibration standards, and QCs were thawed unassisted on ice. Analytes were extracted from the whole blood using protein precipitation with 0.1% (v/v) NH_4OH in ACN spiked with the ISTD **126**. Samples were vortexed for 1 min and then centrifuged at 5590 x *g* for 5 min. Fifteen microlitres of the resulting supernatant, containing the analytes and ISTD, were injected onto the HPLC-MS/MS instrument. Analyte detection for the PK experiments for compounds **49, 49M1, 49M2, 43M1, 47**, and **47M1** was performed on an API 2000 (SCIEX, Toronto, Canada) and on an

API 3200 (SCIEX, Toronto, Canada) for compounds **43** and **43M2**. Each MS/MS instrument was coupled to an Agilent 1100 Series HPLC system (Aligent Technologies, California, US). The unknown analyte concentrations in the experimental PK samples were back-calculated in Analyst software version 1.5.2 (SCIEX, Toronto, Canada) using the respective calibration curve for each analyte.

3.2.6. Non-compartmental pharmacokinetic analysis

GraphPad Prism software version 4 (GraphPad Software Inc., California, US) was used for all statistical analyses and graphic representations. The calculated experimental PK concentrations for the oral and IV groups were used to graph the concentration-time profile for each compound. The mean concentration and error bars, which depicted the standard error of the mean (SEM), were plotted. Additionally, for all oral groups, a logarithm to the base 10 (log_{10}) mean concentration-time profile was plotted against the compound's respective *in vitro Pf*3D7 IC_{50} value, as displayed in **Chapter I, Table 1.1**.

The PK parameters of the compound were determined using NCA in PK Solver, an add-in programme for Microsoft Excel version 16.31 (Microsoft Corporation, Washington, US)[145]. The C_{max} and T_{max} values were directly obtained from the data set. The $T_{½}$ was evaluated during the elimination phase, which was observed when the semilogarithmic plot of the concentration-time profile appeared linear. The $T_{½}$ was determined for the oral and IV groups by calculating the gradient of the curve formed during the terminal phase, which included at least three half-lives of the compound. **Equation 3.1** was applied to calculate the $T_{½}$, where λ is the slope during the terminal phase[118,121,137,141].

$$T_{½} = \frac{\ln(2)}{\lambda}$$ **Equation 3.1**

The $AUC_{0-\infty}$ was calculated for both the oral and IV groups using the linear trapezoidal method, which approximated the integral of the concentration-time curve from zero to infinity[118,121,137,141]. The last experimental time point for each compound differed; therefore, in order to compare exposure values, the curves were integrated to infinity rather than to the last experimental time point.

The Cl and V_d were determined from the IV data. Cl was calculated as shown in **Equation 3.2**, and the Cl values were corrected for mouse weight[118,121,137,141].

$$Cl = \frac{\text{IV dose}}{\text{IV AUC}_{0\text{-}\infty}} \quad \textbf{Equation 3.2}$$

The V_d was calculated according to **Equation 3.3**, where λ is the elimination rate constant, as previously described for **Equation 3.1**[118,121,137,141].

$$V_d = \frac{\text{IV dose}}{\lambda \times \text{IV AUC}_{0\text{-}\infty}} \quad \textbf{Equation 3.3}$$

The percentage F was calculated as shown in **Equation 3.4**[118,121,137,141].

$$F\,(\%) = \frac{\text{IV dose x oral AUC}_{0\text{-}\infty}}{\text{IV AUC}_{0\text{-}\infty}\text{ x oral dose}} \times 100 \quad \textbf{Equation 3.4}$$

The PK parameters are presented as the mean ± SEM. The reported PK data were not corrected for PPB as analytes were quantified in whole blood and, therefore, other blood components, besides plasma, could have contributed to binding. Additionally, the reported *in vitro Pf*3D7 IC_{50} values were not corrected for protein binding in the medium, which is used to culture the malaria parasite, therefore, to keep the comparison consistent between the *in vivo* PK concentrations and the *in vitro* antiplasmodial activities, both parameters were not corrected for the unbound or free fraction and, therefore, the total concentration values are displayed and discussed.

3.3. RESULTS AND DISCUSSION

3.3.1. Review of the bioanalytical method performance

The bioanalytical methods used for the simultaneous quantification of the parent PDBQ, M1, M2, and the ISTD, as described in **Chapter II, Section 2.3.1**, generally performed well, and all analyses fulfilled the criteria that was required to accept the analytical batch, as discussed in **Chapter II, Section 2.1.3.7**. A summary of the HPLC-MS/MS PK analysis for each PDBQ set, including representative chromatograms and statistical data, is presented in **Appendix A**. In summary, no problems were encountered with selectivity and carry over, and the instrument was stable throughout each batch run.

Quadratic regression with a 1/x weighting was used for each analyte's calibration curve, and all fitted curves displayed r values above 0.99. The LLOQ for each analyte was dependent on the instrument sensitivity on the day of analysis, and variabilities were experienced in the analyte LLOQ values across PK batches. All LLOQ concentrations displayed S/N values ≥ 5.

Notably, for the PK analysis of the orally administered preformed **47M1**, the determined LLOQ (62.5 ng/ml) was considerably higher than the LLOQ obtained during method validation (31.3 ng/ml), this was attributed to analyte peak tailing, and therefore, the LLOQ had to be increased to maintain an acceptable S/N value. Nonetheless, this did not have a significant effect on the PK profile of **47M1** as it displayed a concentration of 234 ± 60 ng/ml at the last experimental time point, which was well above the LLOQ. Additionally, analyte peak tailing was observed for the oral and IV PK batches of Set **43**, this was likely as a result of reduced column performance due to extensive use over time. Nonetheless, the determined PK concentrations were accepted since the standards and QCs passed with satisfactory accuracy and precision when automatically integrated.

For each batch, the percentage nominal concentration for the standard and QC samples were within the acceptable range of 85–115%, and the CV values were below 15%, except for the LLOQ where the percentage nominal concentrations were between 80–120%, and the CV values were below 20%[98,101]. Determined concentration values above the limit of quantification (ALOQ) and below the limit of quantification (BLOQ) were excluded from the PK analysis. Furthermore, several concentration values were rationally proposed to be outliers of the dataset and were excluded from the PK analysis. In conclusion, the HPLC-MS/MS analyses were accepted as reliable, accurate, and precise in determining the unknown concentrations of analyte in the whole blood PK study samples. The calculated concentration values for each PK experiment are presented in **Appendix A**. A summary of these results is discussed in the following sections.

3.3.2. Pharmacokinetics of the *ortho*-substituted parent compound 49

Figure 3.2.A displays the whole blood concentration-time profile of **49**, **49M1**, and **49M2** following a single oral administration of 20 mg/kg of **49** to healthy mice. The parent compound and major metabolites were measurable in systemic circulation for up to 10 h post-administration after which the concentrations fell below reliably quantifiable levels. **49M2** was detected as the main metabolite of **49** as it was produced to a greater degree than **49M1**. Both metabolites reached systemic circulation to a greater extent than their parent compound, which could be explained by the extensive metabolic conversion of **49** to **49M1** and **49M2**. **Figure 3.2.B** displays the circulating concentration of each compound in comparison to their respective *in vitro* *Pf*3D7 IC_{50} values. The circulating concentrations of **49M1** and **49M2** were above their respective *Pf*3D7 IC_{50} values (**49M1** = 0.009 μM and **49M2** = 0.019 μM) for 10 h post-administration, but the concentration of **49** fell below its *Pf*3D7 IC_{50} (0.061μM) at 10 h which could indicate a subtherapeutic antimalarial exposure of **49** from 10 h post-administration.

A

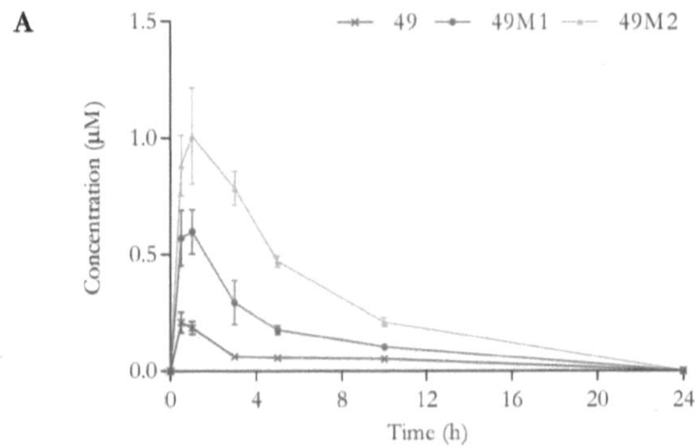

B

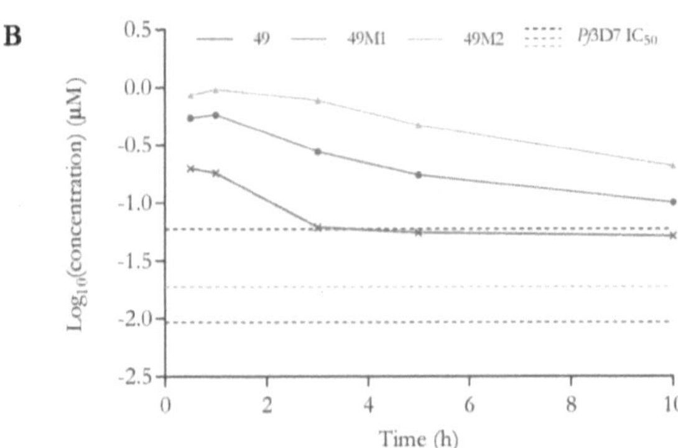

Figure 3.2. Mean (SEM) whole blood **A** concentration-time profile and **B** $\log_{10}$(concentration)-time profile against the *in vitro Pf*3D7 IC_{50} of **49**, **49M1**, and **49M2** following a single oral administration of 20 mg/kg of **49** to healthy mice (*n* = 3).

Figure 3.3 displays the whole blood concentration-time profile of **49** following a single IV administration of 5 mg/kg of **49** to healthy mice. The major metabolites of **49** were undetectable at concentrations above each analyte's respective LLOQ of 31.3 ng/ml (data not shown).

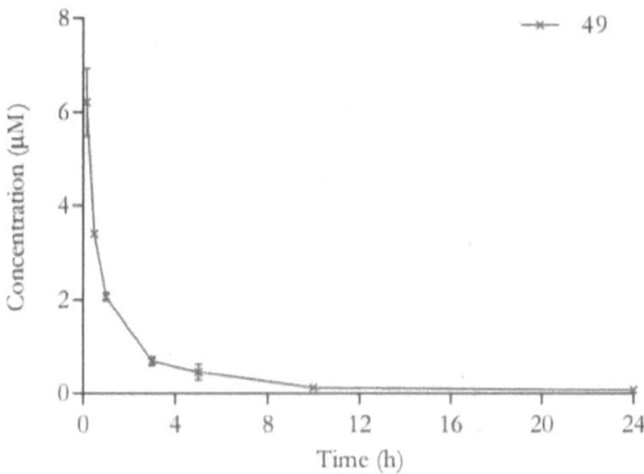

Figure 3.3. Mean (SEM) whole blood concentration-time profile of **49** following a single IV administration of 5 mg/kg of **49** to healthy mice ($n = 3$). Metabolites were undetectable at levels above their respective LLOQ concentration.

Table 3.3 presents a summary of the PK parameters of **49**, **49M1**, and **49M2** following single oral and IV administrations of the parent **49** to healthy mice. **49M2** reached the highest maximal concentration of 1.1 ± 0.1 µM, followed by **49M1** with a C_{max} of 0.6 ± 0.1 µM and last the parent **49**, which displayed the lowest initial systemic absorption with a C_{max} of 0.22 ± 0.04 µM. The rate of systemic absorption of **49** and **49M1** was rapid, exhibited by similar T_{max} values of 0.7 ± 0.2 and 0.8 ± 0.2 h, respectively. **49M2** displayed a relatively slower systemic absorption achieving a T_{max} value of 1.7 ± 0.7 h, which could be an indication of a slight delay in the formation of **49M2** in the liver. The $T_{1/2}$ of **49** was similar after oral and IV administration with moderate elimination half-lives of 4 ± 1 and 5.1 ± 0.9 h, respectively. The metabolites displayed $T_{1/2}$ values comparable to the parent of 4.4 ± 0.5 h for **49M1** and 3.9 ± 0.7 h for **49M2**. **49** exhibited a high *in vitro* Cl_{int} of 1224 ml/min/kg, however, in an *in vivo* setting, **49** demonstrated a low Cl of 0.6 ± 0.1 ml/min/kg. Due to the highly lipophilic nature of **49**, the observed low *in vivo* Cl could be attributed to high PPB; this can be corroborated by determining the *in vitro* PPB of **49**[77]. **49** had a low V_d of 0.25 ± 0.04 l/kg indicating that the majority of **49** was present in circulation and further substantiating the conjecture that the low Cl of **49** could be in part due to high PPB. Besides high PPB, the observed low Cl and low V_d of **49** could also be as a result of **49** being sequestered within the murine blood cells, an occurrence that has been demonstrated with CQ, which is also a weakly basic drug[146]. Following this hypothesis, the absence of the major metabolites in circulation after IV administration of **49** could be explained by the restriction of **49** in the murine blood cell which, therefore, makes the parent unavailable for systemic metabolism. **49** displayed poor oral exposure as shown by its relatively low $AUC_{0-\infty}$ of 1.1 ± 0.1 μM.h, **49M1** and **49M2** displayed a greater exposure of 3.1 ± 0.3 and 6.7 ± 0.3 μM.h, respectively. The exposure of the metabolites exceeded that of their parent with a 2.8-fold difference in the $AUC_{0-\infty}$ of **49M1** to **49** and a 6.1-fold difference in the $AUC_{0-\infty}$ of **49M2** to **49**. Furthermore, the biotransformation of **49** to **49M2** was higher than that of **49** to **49M1** as indicated by a 2.1-fold difference in the $AUC_{0-\infty}$ of **49M2** compared to **49M1**. F of **49** was poor, with a value of 2.2%.

Table 3.3. Non-compartmental PK parameters of **49**, **49M1**, and **49M2** following single oral and IV administrations of 20 and 5 mg/kg, respectively of **49** to healthy mice

PK parameter[a]	**Oral**[b]			**IV**[b]
	49	**49M1**	**49M2**	**49**
C_{max} (μM)	0.22 ± 0.04	0.6 ± 0.1	1.1 ± 0.1	-
T_{max} (h)	0.7 ± 0.2	0.8 ± 0.2	1.7 ± 0.7	-
$T_{1/2}$ (h)	4 ± 1	4.4 ± 0.5	3.9 ± 0.7	5.1 ± 0.9
Cl (ml/min/kg)	-	-	-	0.6 ± 0.1
V_d (l/kg)	-	-	-	0.25 ± 0.04
$AUC_{0-\infty}$ (μM.h)	1.1 ± 0.1	3.1 ± 0.3	6.7 ± 0.3	12 ± 1
F (%)	2.2	-	-	-

[a]Values reported as the mean ± SEM. [b]*n* = 3.

3.3.3. Pharmacokinetics of the *ortho*-substituted metabolite 49M1

Figure 3.4.A displays the whole blood concentration-time profile of **49M1** following a single oral administration of 20 mg/kg of preformed **49M1** to healthy mice. **49M1** was detected for up to 24 h after administration. As shown in **Figure 3.4.B**, the circulating concentration of **49M1** remained above its *Pf*3D7 IC_{50} (0.009 μM) for 24 h post-administration. Furthermore, the concentration of **49M1** at the 24 h time point was 16.3-fold higher than its *Pf*3D7 IC_{50}, which could promote sustained antimalarial exposure. The whole blood concentration-time data of **49M1** following an IV administration of 5 mg/kg of preformed **49M1** to healthy mice is presented in **Appendix A, Table A.4**.

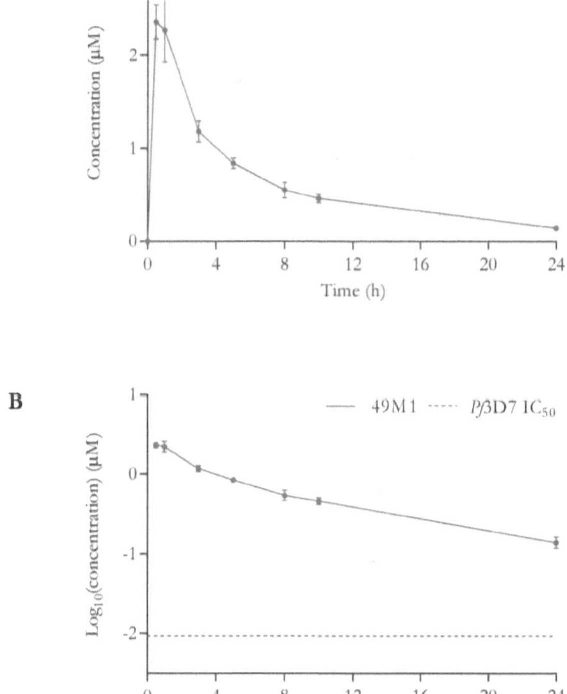

Figure 3.4. Mean (SEM) whole blood **A** concentration-time profile and **B** $\log_{10}$(concentration)-time profile against the *in vitro* *Pf*3D7 IC_{50} of **49M1** following a single oral administration of 20 mg/kg of preformed **49M1** to healthy mice ($n = 3$).

Table 3.4 displays a summary of the PK parameters of **49M1** following single oral and IV administrations of preformed **49M1** to healthy mice. **49M1** was rapidly absorbed with a C_{max} value of 2.4 ± 0.3 μM and a T_{max} value of 0.7 ± 0.2 h. The similar T_{max} values of **49M1** that were obtained when preformed **49M1** was administered and when its parent was administered (**49M1** T_{max} = 0.8 ± 0.2 h) suggests a fast conversion of **49** to **49M1**. **49M1** displayed a relatively long $T_{1/2}$ of 8.21 ± 0.05 h after oral administration and 12.2 ± 0.5 h after IV administration. **49M1** had a low Cl of 0.49 ± 0.03 ml/min/kg and a low V_d of 0.51 ± 0.01 l/kg. The $AUC_{0\text{-}\infty}$ of **49M1** following the oral administration was 16 ± 2 μM.h, and the F was 22.2%. **49M1** demonstrated a higher oral absorption than **49**, as shown by its higher F compared to that of **49** (F = 2.2%). The exposure of **49M1** was higher when preformed **49M1** was administered compared to when it was administered as the parent. This is illustrated by a 5.2-fold increase in the oral $AUC_{0\text{-}\infty}$ of **49M1** when preformed **49M1** was administered compared to when **49** was administered (**49M1** $AUC_{0\text{-}\infty}$ = 3.1 ± 0.3 μM.h). Furthermore, the C_{max} of **49M1** was higher, and the $T_{1/2}$ was longer when the preformed metabolite was administered compared to that obtained when the parent was administered (**49M1** C_{max} = 0.6 ± 0.1 μM and **49M1** $T_{1/2}$ = 4.4 ± 0.5 h). These observations signify that the preformed metabolite was able to reach and maintain higher concentrations than the parent and its formed metabolites.

Table 3.4. Non-compartmental PK parameters of **49M1** following single oral and IV administrations of 20 and 5 mg/kg, respectively of **49M1** to healthy mice

PK parameter[a]	**49M1**	
	Oral[b]	**IV**[b]
C_{max} (µM)	2.4 ± 0.3	-
T_{max} (h)	0.7 ± 0.2	-
$T_{1/2}$ (h)	8.21 ± 0.05	12.2 ± 0.5
Cl (ml/min/kg)	-	0.49 ± 0.03
V_d (l/kg)	-	0.51 ± 0.01
$AUC_{0-\infty}$ (µM.h)	16 ± 2	18 ± 1
F (%)	22.2	-

[a]Values reported as the mean ± SEM. [b]*n* = 3.

3.3.4. Pharmacokinetics of the *ortho*-substituted metabolite 49M2

Figure 3.5.A displays the concentration-time profile of **49M2** following a single oral administration of 20 mg/kg of preformed **49M2** to healthy mice. As observed with orally administered preformed **49M1, 49M2** was also detected for 24 h following administration. In **Figure 3.5.B**, the circulating concentration of **49M2** remained above its *Pf*3D7 IC_{50} (0.019 µM) for 24 h post-oral administration. Additionally, at the 24 h time point, the concentration of **49M2** was 8.7-fold higher than its *Pf*3D7 IC_{50}, which could contribute towards sustained antimalarial exposure. The concentration-time data of **49M2** following an IV administration of 5 mg/kg of preformed **49M2** to healthy mice is presented in **Appendix A, Table A.10**.

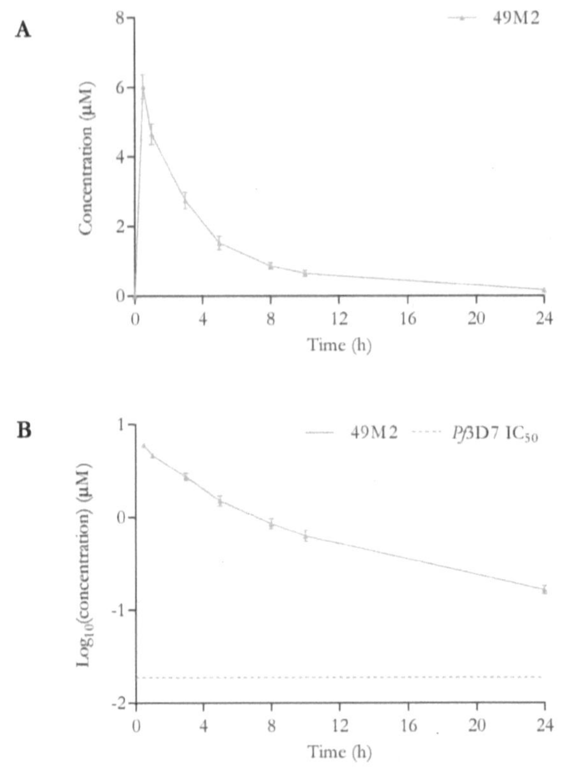

Figure 3.5. Mean (SEM) whole blood **A** concentration-time profile and **B** $\log_{10}$(concentration)-time profile against the *in vitro* *Pf*3D7 IC_{50} of **49M2** following a single oral administration of 20 mg/kg of preformed **49M2** to healthy mice (n = 3).

Table 3.5 displays a summary of the PK parameters of **49M2** following single oral and IV administrations of preformed **49M2** to healthy mice. The C_{max} and T_{max} of **49M2** were 6.0 ± 0.5 µM and 0.5 h, respectively, indicating high and rapid oral absorption. The absorption of **49M2** was faster when the preformed metabolite was administered compared to its systemic absorption when the parent was administered (**49M2** T_{max} = 1.7 ± 0.7 h), this could be a result of a slow or delayed conversion and release of **49** to **49M2**. The oral and IV $T_{1/2}$ were moderate and similar, with $T_{1/2}$ values of 7.0 ± 0.7 and 6.6 ± 0.6 h, respectively. The Cl of 0.35 ± 0.02 ml/min/kg was slow, and the V_d of 0.20 ± 0.01 l/kg was low. **49M2** had a relatively high oral exposure of 28 ± 1 µM.h and a low to moderate F of 28.1%.

Preformed **49M2** displayed a 5.5-fold higher C_{max} compared to the C_{max} reached when it was administered as the parent (**49M2** C_{max} = 1.1 ± 0.1 μM). Additionally, **49M2** displayed a longer $T_{1/2}$ when administered directly as the metabolite compared to when it was administered as the parent (**49M2** $T_{1/2}$ = 3.9 ± 0.7 h). And lastly, a 4.2-fold increase in the oral exposure of **49M2** was exhibited when the preformed metabolite was administered compared to that when the parent was administered (**49M2** $AUC_{0-\infty}$ = 6.7 ± 0.3 μM.h). Similar observations were seen when comparing preformed **49M1** to the parent **49**. Preformed **49M2** reached a 2.5-fold higher C_{max} than preformed **49M1** (C_{max} = 2.4 ± 0.3 μM). Preformed **49M1** and **49M2** displayed similar $T_{1/2}$, but their oral exposures differed as **49M2** showed a 1.8-fold higher $AUC_{0-\infty}$ compared to that of **49M1** ($AUC_{0-\infty}$ = 16 ± 2 μM.h). Although the overall exposure of preformed **49M2** was higher than that of preformed **49M1**, the extent of oral absorption of **49M1** and **49M2** was similar as they both presented comparable F values. Nonetheless, **49M2** displayed a more favourable PK profile based upon on its higher C_{max} and greater $AUC_{0-\infty}$ values, compared to **49M1**.

Table 3.5. Non-compartmental PK parameters of **49M2** following single oral and IV administrations of 20 and 5 mg/kg, respectively of **49M2** to healthy mice

PK parameter[a]	49M2	
	Oral[b]	IV[b]
C_{max} (μM)	6.0 ± 0.5	-
T_{max} (h)	0.5	-
$T_{1/2}$ (h)	7.0 ± 0.7	6.6 ± 0.6
Cl (ml/min/kg)	-	0.35 ± 0.02
V_d (l/kg)	-	0.20 ± 0.01
$AUC_{0-\infty}$ (μM.h)	28 ± 1	27 ± 1
F (%)	28.1	-

[a]Values reported as the mean ± SEM. [b]*n* = 3.

3.3.5. Pharmacokinetics of the *meta*-substituted parent 43

Figure 3.6.A displays the whole blood concentration-time profile of **43, 43M1**, and **43M2** following an oral administration of 20 mg/kg of **43** to healthy mice. **43** was detected in the blood for up to 5 h post-administration, and **43M1** and **43M2** were detected in the blood for up to 10 h following administration after which, the circulating concentrations fell below their respective LLOQ values. As shown in **Figure 3.6.B**, the observed concentrations of the parent and metabolites remained above each analyte's *Pf*3D7 IC_{50} (**43** = 0.038 μM, **43M1** = 0.016 μM, and **43M2** = 0.036 μM) for only a relatively short period of time, which could result in a limited duration of antimalarial activity.

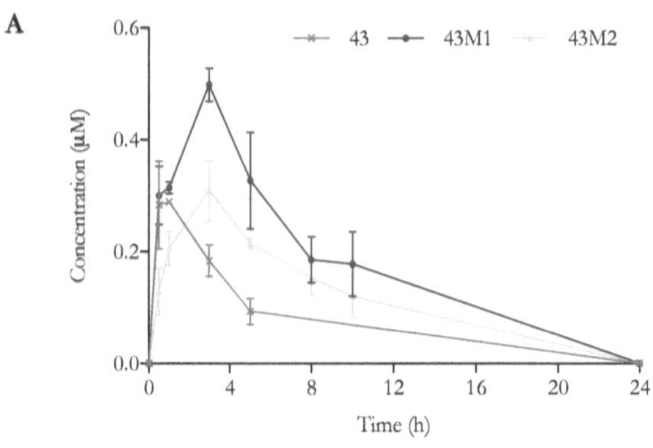

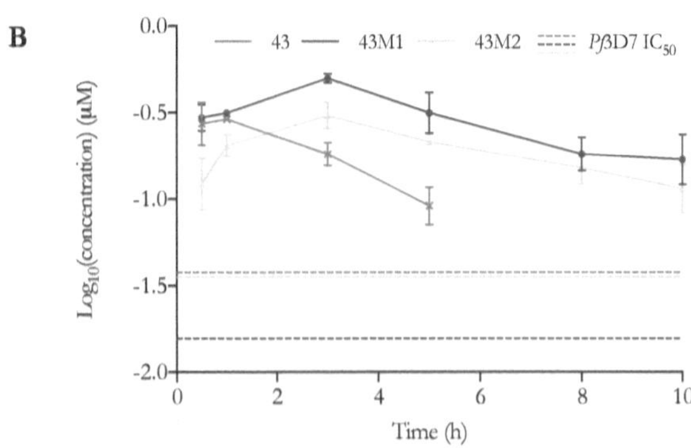

Figure 3.6. Mean (SEM) whole blood **A** concentration-time profile and **B** $\log_{10}$(concentration)-time profile against the *in vitro Pf*3D7 IC_{50} of **43, 43M1**, and **43M2** following a single oral administration of 20 mg/kg of **43** to healthy mice ($n = 2$).

Figure 3.7 displays the whole blood concentration-time profile of **43** following an IV administration of 5 mg/kg of **43** to healthy mice. Compound **43** was detectable for 10 h post-IV administration, however, the major metabolites of **43** could not be detected at levels above their respective LLOQ of 15.1 ng/ml (data not shown). This suggests that **43M1** and **43M2** are products of first-pass metabolism, a similar finding to that observed for **49**. **43** was observed for 5 h longer after IV administration compared to oral administration, which could likely be a result of a significantly larger initial concentration of **43** being introduced directly into systemic circulation; moreover, the HPLC-MS/MS method was not sensitive enough to detect the lower levels present in the oral group after 5 h.

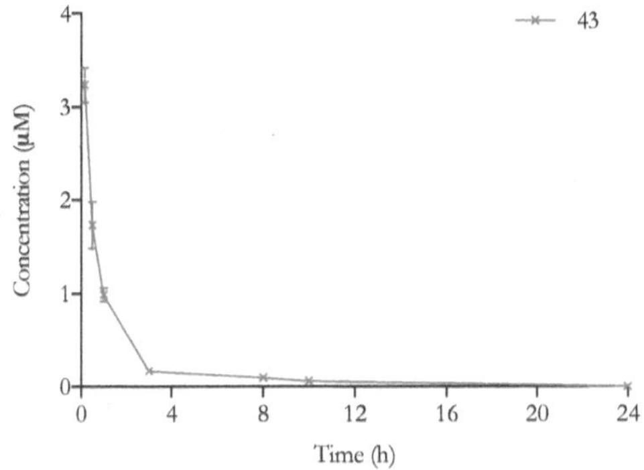

Figure 3.7. Mean (SEM) whole blood concentration-time profile of **43** following a single IV administration of 5 mg/kg of **43** to healthy mice (n = 2). Metabolites were undetectable at levels above their respective LLOQ concentrations.

Table 3.6 displays a summary of the PK parameters of **43**, **43M1**, and **43M2** following single oral and IV administrations of the parent **43** to healthy mice. **43M1** reached the highest C_{max} of 0.50 ± 0.02 μM, and **43** and **43M2** showed similar C_{max} values of 0.32 ± 0.04 and 0.31 ± 0.05 μM, respectively. **43** displayed rapid absorption with a T_{max} value of 0.8 ± 0.3 h, whereas both metabolites showed relatively slow systemic absorption with the same T_{max} value of 3.0 h. **43** had a short $T_{1/2}$ of 2.5 ± 0.5 h, whereas the metabolites displayed a relatively longer $T_{1/2}$ of 5.2 ± 0.2 and 7 ± 3 h for **43M1** and **43M2**, respectively. **43** exhibited a low Cl of 1.574 ± 0.007 ml/min/kg however, this was 2.6-fold higher than the Cl of **49** (0.6 ± 0.1 ml/min/kg). **43** was largely dispersed in systemic circulation, as displayed by its relatively low V_d of 0.4 ± 0.2 l/kg. **43** was poorly absorbed as shown by its relatively low C_{max} and low oral $AUC_{0-\infty}$ of 1.3 ± 0.3 μM.h. Furthermore, **43** displayed a low IV exposure, with an $AUC_{0-\infty}$ of 4.38 ± 0.02 μM.h, compared to the IV $AUC_{0-\infty}$ of **49** (12 ± 1 μM.h); this could likely be attributed to the relatively higher Cl of **43** compared to **49.** The metabolites of **43** were better systemically absorbed than the parent, **43M1** showed the greatest exposure of 4.4 ± 0.9 μM.h, followed by **43M2** with an exposure of 3 ± 1 μM.h. The oral exposures of **43M1** and **43M2** were 3.4- and 2.3-fold higher, respectively, than the exposure of **43**. The comparable $AUC_{0-\infty}$ and T_{max} values of **43M1** and **43M2** suggests that they encountered similar extents of metabolism and subsequent absorption. **43** displayed a low F of 7.5%. As proposed for **49**, the absence of the major metabolites in circulation after IV administration of **43** could possibly be due to high PPB and accumulation of **43** within the murine blood cell which resulted in the parent being unavailable for systemic metabolism. This hypothesis correlates with the low Cl and low V_d of **43**, however, mouse PPB and drug accumulation studies, within the murine red blood cell, will need to be performed to support this theory. In general, after oral administration of **43**, the parents and major metabolites did not exhibit any improved PK properties compared to that of **49**, **49M1**, and **49M2** after **49** was orally administered.

Table 3.6. Non-compartmental PK parameters of **43**, **43M1**, and **43M2** following single oral and IV administrations of 20 and 5 mg/kg, respectively of **43** to healthy mice

PK parameter[a]	**Oral**[b]			**IV**[b]
	43	**43M1**	**43M2**	**43**
C_{max} (µM)	0.32 ± 0.04	0.50 ± 0.02	0.31 ± 0.05	-
T_{max} (h)	0.8 ± 0.3	3.0	3.0	-
$T_{1/2}$ (h)	2.5 ± 0.5	5.2 ± 0.2	7 ± 3	3 ± 1
Cl (ml/min/kg)	-	-	-	1.574 ± 0.007
V_d (l/kg)	-	-	-	0.4 ± 0.2
$AUC_{0-\infty}$ (µM.h)	1.3 ± 0.3	4.4 ± 0.9	3 ± 1	4.38 ± 0.02
F (%)	7.5	-	-	-

[a]Values reported as the mean ± SEM. [b]*n* = 2.

3.3.6. Pharmacokinetics of the *meta*-substituted metabolite 43M1

Figure 3.8.A shows the whole blood concentration-time profile of **43M1** following an oral administration of 20 mg/kg of preformed **43M1** to healthy mice. **43M1** was detectable for 24 h post-administration and the circulating concentration of **43M1** at the 24 h time point was 10.5-fold higher than its *Pf*3D7 IC_{50} (0.016 µM), which could reflect a high sustained antimalarial exposure of **43M1** for up to 24 h post-administration, as shown in **Figure 3.8.B**. The whole blood concentration-time data of preformed **43M1** following IV administration to healthy mice is presented in **Appendix A, Table A.20**.

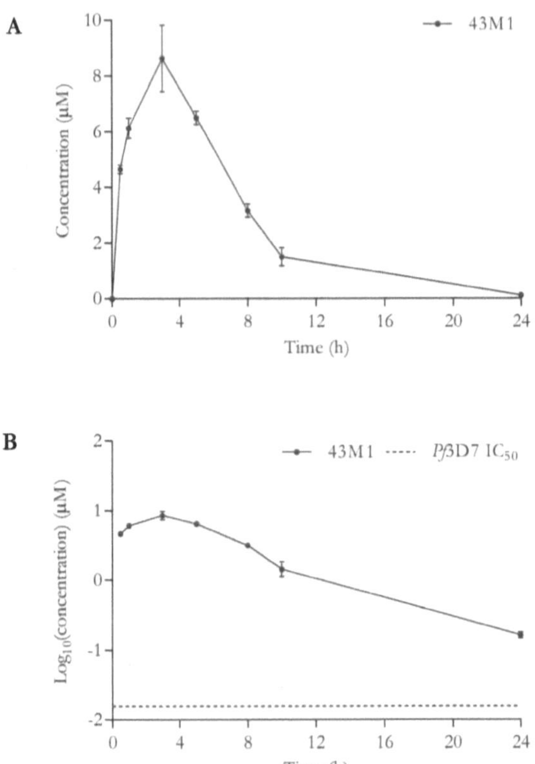

Figure 3.8. Mean (SEM) whole blood **A** concentration-time profile and **B** $\log_{10}$(concentration)-time profile against the *in vitro Pf*3D7 IC_{50} of **43M1** following a single oral administration of 20 mg/kg of preformed **43M1** to healthy mice (*n* = 3).

Table 3.7 displays a summary of the PK parameters of **43M1** following single oral and IV administrations of preformed **43M1** to healthy mice. **43M1** reached a relatively high C_{max} of 8 ± 1 μM, and this was achieved relatively slowly with a T_{max} of 3.7 ± 0.7 h. The T_{max} of **43M1** when preformed **43M1** was administered is comparable to that when its parent **43** was administered (**43M1** T_{max} = 3.0 h). This suggests a fast conversion of **43** to **43M1**, but a slow release of **43M1** from the liver into systemic circulation. **43M1** displayed a moderate $T_{1/2}$ of 3.6 ± 0.4 h, a slow Cl of 0.245 ± 0.002 ml/min/kg, and a low V_d of 0.12 ± 0.03 l/kg. **43M1** attained a relatively high exposure with an oral $AUC_{0-\infty}$ of 62 ± 3 μM.h and a relatively high F of 42.3%. **43M1** exhibited a higher F than **43** (F = 7.5%). The oral exposure of **43M1** was higher when administered as preformed **43M1**, rather than when its parent **43** was administered (**43M1** $AUC_{0-\infty}$ = 4.4 ± 0.9 µM.h), as shown by the 14.1-fold increase in the $AUC_{0-\infty}$ of preformed **43M1** compared to formed **43M1**. Additionally, a 16.0-fold increase in the C_{max} of **43M1** was observed when administered as the metabolite compared to when **43M1** was administered as the parent. Lastly, **43M1** exhibited higher C_{max}, oral $AUC_{0-\infty}$, and F values than that of preformed **49M1** (C_{max} = 2.4 ± 0.3 µM, $AUC_{0-\infty}$ = 16 ± 2 µM.h, and F = 22.2%), and preformed **49M2** (C_{max} = 6.0 ± 0.5 µM, $AUC_{0-\infty}$ = 28 ± 1 µM.h, and F = 28.1%), which suggests that **43M1** could display greater antimalarial activity than **49M1** or **49M2** as it is able to attain higher levels *in vivo.*

Table 3.7. Non-compartmental PK parameters of **43M1** following single oral and IV administrations of 20 and 5 mg/kg, respectively of **43M1** to healthy mice

PK parameter[a]	43M1	
	Oral[b]	IV[c]
C_{max} (µM)	8 ± 1	-
T_{max} (h)	3.7 ± 0.7	-
$T_{1/2}$ (h)	3.6 ± 0.4	6 ± 1
Cl (ml/min/kg)	-	0.245 ± 0.002
V_d (l/kg)	-	0.12 ± 0.03
$AUC_{0-\infty}$ (µM.h)	62 ± 3	36.4 ± 0.3
F (%)	42.3	-

[a]Values reported as the mean ± SEM. [b]*n* = 3. [c]*n* = 2 (animal lost during the anaesthesia procedure).

3.3.7. Pharmacokinetics of the *meta*-substituted metabolite 43M2

Figure 3.9.A shows the whole blood concentration-time profile of **43M2** following an oral administration of 20 mg/kg of preformed **43M2** to healthy mice. **43M2** was detected for only 10 h post-administration, although it was present at low concentrations beyond the 10 h time point, these concentrations could not be reliably quantified as they were below the LLOQ. However, for up to 10 h following administration, the circulating concentration of **43M2** remained above its *Pf*3D7 IC_{50} (0.036 μM), as shown in **Figure 3.9.B**. The mean whole blood concentration-time data of **43M2** following an IV administration of preformed **43M2** to healthy mice is presented in **Appendix A, Table A.24**.

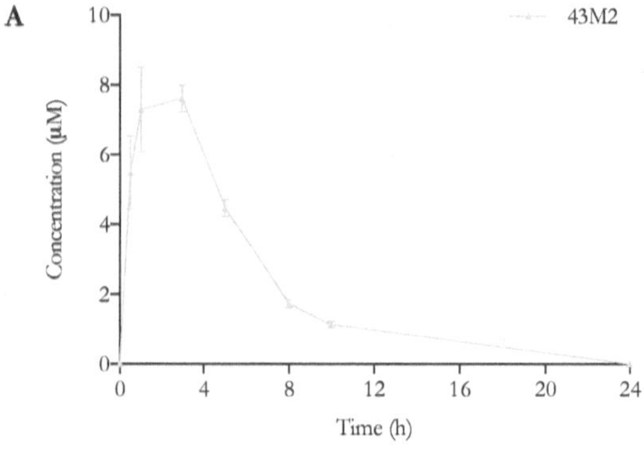

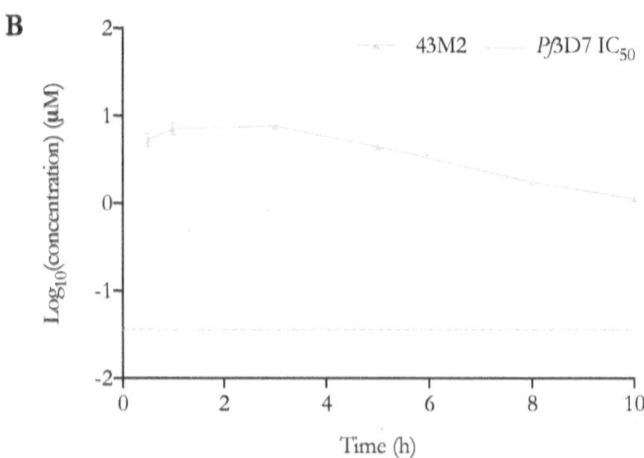

Figure 3.9. Mean (SEM) whole blood **A** concentration-time profile and **B** log_{10}(concentration)-time profile against the *in vitro Pf*3D7 IC_{50} of **43M2** following a single oral administration of 20 mg/kg of preformed **43M2** to healthy mice (n = 3).

Table 3.8 displays a summary of the PK parameters of **43M2** following single oral and IV administrations of preformed **43M2** to healthy mice. **43M2** reached a peak concentration of 8.5 ± 0.5 μM, and this was achieved relatively slowly, as shown by the T_{max} value of 2.3 ± 0.7 h. **43M2** displayed a relatively short $T_{1/2}$ of 3.2 ± 0.3 h, which could be an underprediction of the true $T_{1/2}$ as the elimination phase was not fully represented in the PK analysis. The Cl of **43M2** was slow at 0.209 ± 0.008 ml/min/kg and the V_d was low at 0.065 ± 0.005 l/kg. **43M2** exhibited a relatively high oral exposure with an $AUC_{0-\infty}$ of 51 ± 2 μM.h and a low to moderate F of 25.1%. **43M2** displayed a higher F than **43** (F = 7.5%). When **43M2** was administered as the preformed metabolite, it displayed a 27.4-fold increase in its C_{max} and a 17.0-fold increase in its $AUC_{0-\infty}$ compared to when it was administered as the parent (**43M2** C_{max} = 0.31 ± 0.05 μM and **43M2** $AUC_{0-\infty}$ = 3 ± 1 μM.h). The F of preformed **43M2** was similar to that of preformed **49M1** (F = 22.2%) and preformed **49M2** (F = 28.1%). However, the C_{max} and overall exposure of preformed **43M2** was higher than that of preformed **49M1** (C_{max} = 2.4 ± 0.3 μM and $AUC_{0-\infty}$ = 16 ± 2 μM.h) and preformed **49M2** (C_{max} = 6.0 ± 0.5 μM and $AUC_{0-\infty}$ = 28 ± 1 μM.h), which suggests that **43M2** could demonstrate greater antimalarial exposure, compared to **49M1** and **49M2**. Lastly, preformed **43M2** and **43M1** displayed equivalent C_{max} values, but **43M2** exhibited a 0.8-fold lower $AUC_{0-\infty}$ than the $AUC_{0-\infty}$ of **43M1** (62 ± 3 μM.h); and their F values differed, where **43M2** displayed a 0.6-fold lower F than **43M1** (F = 42.3%). As shown in **Chapter I, Table 1.1**, the *in vitro Pf*3D7 IC_{50} values demonstrate that **43M1** is 2.3 times more active than **43M2** which suggests that, although **43M2** displayed a favourable PK profile, **43M1** might deliver higher *in vivo* antimalarial activity since it is more potent and displayed greater oral exposure compared to **43M2**.

Table 3.8. Non-compartmental PK parameters of **43M2** following single oral and IV administrations of 20 and 5 mg/kg, respectively of **43M2** to healthy mice

PK parameter[a]	**43M2**	
	Oral[b]	**IV**[b]
C_{max} (μM)	8.5 ± 0.5	-
T_{max} (h)	2.3 ± 0.7	-
$T_{1/2}$ (h)	3.2 ± 0.3	3.6 ± 0.2
Cl (ml/min/kg)	-	0.209 ± 0.008
V_d (l/kg)	-	0.065 ± 0.005
$AUC_{0-\infty}$ (μM.h)	51 ± 2	45 ± 2
F (%)	25.1	-

[a]Values reported as the mean ± SEM. [b]*n* = 3.

3.3.8. Pharmacokinetics of the *para*-substituted parent compound 47

Figure 3.10.A displays the whole blood concentration-time profile of **47**, **47M1**, and **47M2** following a single oral administration of 20 mg/kg of **47** to healthy mice. **47** and **47M2** were detected in the blood for up to 10 h post-administration, and **47M1** was detected for up to 24 h post-administration. As shown in **Figure 3.10.B**, the circulating concentrations of **47** and **47M1** were above their respective *in vitro Pf*3D7 IC_{50} (**47** = 0.033 μM and **47M1** = 0.013 μM) for the duration of time in which they were detectable; however, **47M2** did not attain concentrations above its relatively high *Pf*3D7 IC_{50} (0.291 μM) throughout the experimental time course. The oral concentration-time profile of **47** differs to that of the other parents **49** and **43** (**Figure 3.2** and **Figure 3.6**, respectively), in that the parent **47** displayed a relatively high initial absorption compared to the formed metabolites **47M1** and **47M2**, and this was not exhibited in the PK profiles **49** and **43**. Furthermore, **47M1** was detected for up to 24 h following administration, and this was also not observed for any other metabolites that were produced after parent administration, as they were only measurable for up to 10 h post-administration.

A

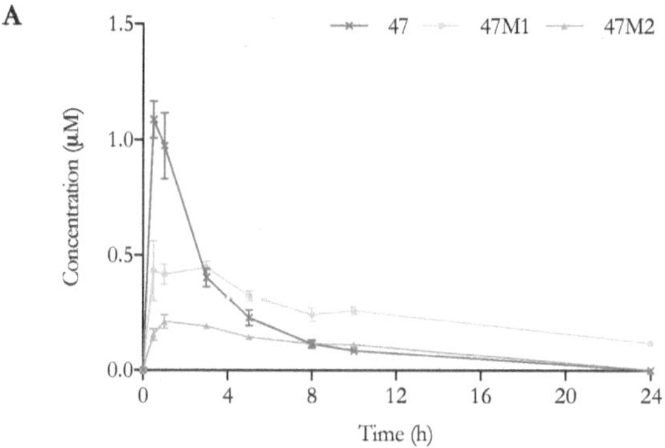

B

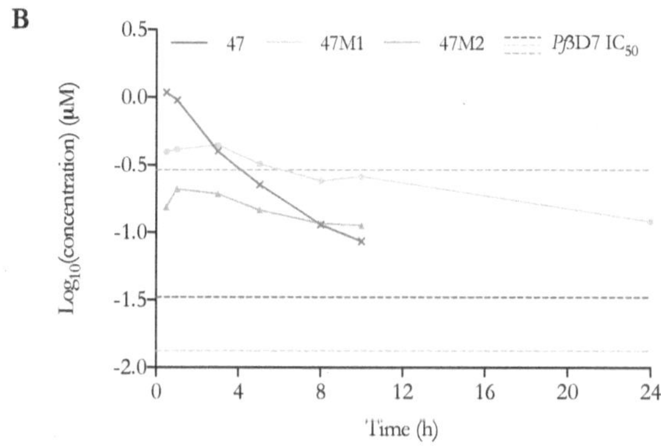

Figure 3.10. Mean (SEM) whole blood **A** concentration-time profile and **B** log_{10}(concentration)-time profile against the *in vitro Pf*3D7 IC_{50} of **47**, **47M1**, and **47M2** following a single oral administration of 20 mg/kg of **47** to healthy mice (n = 3).

Figure 3.11 shows the concentration-time profile of **47** following an IV administration of 5 mg/kg of **47** to healthy mice. The major metabolites of **47** could not be detected in the blood at levels above their respective LLOQ value of 31.3 ng/ml (data not shown).

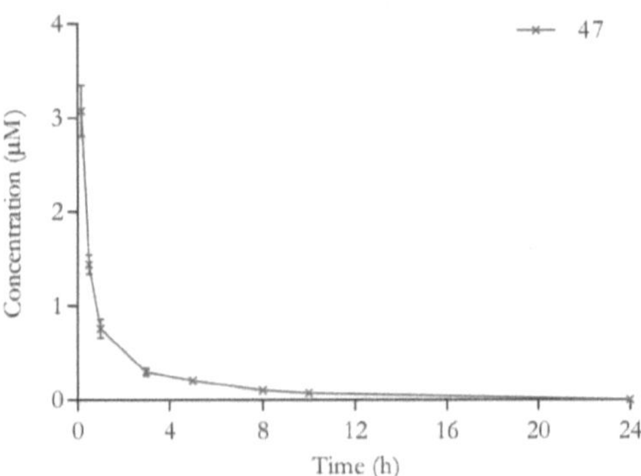

Figure 3.11. Mean (SEM) whole blood concentration-time profile of **47** following a single IV administration of 5 mg/kg of **47** to healthy mice (n = 3). Metabolites were undetectable at levels above their respective LLOQ concentrations.

Table 3.9 displays a summary of the PK parameters of **47**, **47M1**, and **47M2** following single oral and IV administrations of **47** to healthy mice. The parent **47** reached the highest C_{max} of 1.09 ± 0.03 μM and displayed rapid absorption with a T_{max} value of 0.7 ± 0.2 h, compared to **47M1** and **47M2** which displayed peak concentrations of 0.54 ± 0.07 and 0.23 ± 0.02 μM and T_{max} values of 2.2 ± 0.8 and 1.7 ± 0.7 h, respectively. The metabolites displayed a slower movement from the liver to systemic circulation and did not reach C_{max} concentrations as high as **47**. **47** displayed a short $T_{1/2}$ of 3.4 ± 0.5 h, whereas **47M1** and **47M2** exhibited relatively longer $T_{1/2}$ of 14 ± 2 and 11 ± 1 h, respectively. **47** had a low Cl of 1.5 ± 0.1 ml/min/kg, and a low V_d of 0.4 ± 0.1 l/kg. As observed with **49** and **43**, after IV administration of the parent, the major metabolites were undetectable in circulation. Given the low Cl and low V_d of **47**, it is proposed that the parent is restricted in the blood cell or highly protein bound which, therefore, protected the parent from systemic metabolism. Although **47** exhibited the highest C_{max}, it displayed a comparatively low oral exposure with an $AUC_{0-\infty}$ of 3.93 ± 0.05 μM.h; this can most likely be ascribed to its short $T_{1/2}$. **47M1** displayed the highest exposure with an $AUC_{0-\infty}$ of 8.4 ± 0.4 μM.h, and **47M2** displayed the lowest exposure of 3.3 ± 0.1 μM.h. **47** reached the highest F of 24.6% compared to the other parents, **49** (F = 2.2%) and **43** (F = 7.5%). F of **47** was comparable to that of several preformed metabolites, specifically **49M1** (F = 22.2%), **49M2** (F = 28.1%), and **43M2** (F = 25.1%).

Table 3.9. Non-compartmental PK parameters of **47**, **47M1**, and **47M2** following single oral and IV administrations of 20 and 5 mg/kg, respectively of **47** to healthy mice

PK parameter[a]	**Oral**[b]			**IV**[b]
	47	**47M1**	**47M2**	**47**
C_{max} (μM)	1.09 ± 0.03	0.54 ± 0.07	0.23 ± 0.02	-
T_{max} (h)	0.7 ± 0.2	2.2 ± 0.8	1.7 ± 0.7	-
$T_{1/2}$ (h)	3.4 ± 0.5	14 ± 2	11 ± 1	3.1 ± 0.7
Cl (ml/min/kg)	-	-	-	1.5 ± 0.1
V_d (l/kg)	-	-	-	0.4 ± 0.1
$AUC_{0-\infty}$ (μM.h)	3.93 ± 0.05	8.4 ± 0.4	3.3 ± 0.1	4.6 ± 0.3
F (%)	24.6	-	-	-

[a]Values reported as the mean ± SEM. [b]*n* = 3.

3.3.9. Pharmacokinetics of the *para*-substituted metabolite 47M1

Figure 3.12.A displays the whole blood concentration-time profile of **47M1** following a single 20 mg/kg oral administration of preformed **47M1** to mice. As shown in **Figure 3.12.B, 47M1** was detected for up to 24 h post-administration. Furthermore, the circulating concentration of **47M1** at the 24 h time point was 57.9-fold higher than its *Pf*3D7 IC_{50} (0.013 μM); this could promote potent and sustained antimalarial activity for up to 24 h post-administration. The whole blood concentration-time data of **47M1** following IV administration of preformed **47M1** to healthy mice is presented in **Appendix A, Table A.30**.

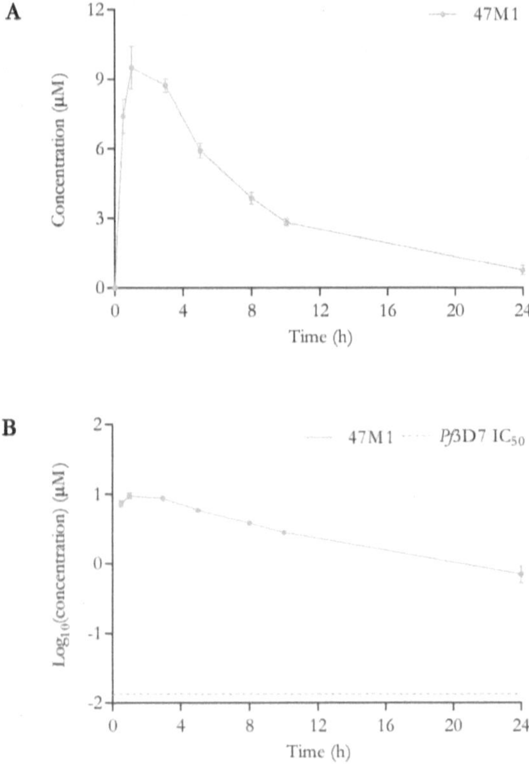

Figure 3.12. Mean (SEM) whole blood **A** concentration-time profile and **B** log_{10}(concentration)-time profile against the *in vitro Pf*3D7 IC_{50} of **47M1** following a single oral administration of 20 mg/kg of preformed **47M1** to healthy mice (n = 3).

Table 3.10 displays a summary of the PK parameters of **47M1** following single oral and IV administrations of preformed **47M1** to healthy mice. **47M1** reached the highest peak concentration of 9.4 ± 0.5 μM in 1.7 ± 0.8 h compared to all the other preformed metabolites, where the second-highest C_{max} obtained was 8 ± 1 μM by **43M1**, and the lowest C_{max} was 2.4 ± 0.3 μM from **49M1**. **47M1** displayed a moderate oral $T_{1/2}$ of 7 ± 1 h and a slow Cl and low V_d of 0.15 ± 0.02 ml/min/kg and 0.10 ± 0.02 l/kg, respectively. Preformed **47M1** displayed a shorter $T_{1/2}$ compared to that observed when it was administered as **47** (**47M1** $T_{1/2}$ = 14 ± 2 h), this could be as a result of the elimination phase being underrepresented during the PK analysis of preformed **47M1**. **47M1** exhibited a relatively high oral exposure with an $AUC_{0-\infty}$ of 93 ± 9 μM.h. This was the highest oral exposure attained compared to the other preformed metabolites whose $AUC_{0-\infty}$ values ranged between 16 ± 2 μM.h for **49M1** to 62 ± 3 μM.h for **43M1**. Although **47M1** displayed the highest exposure and C_{max} compared to the other preformed metabolites, it showed a similar F to that of **43M1** (F = 42.3%). **47M1** reached a 17.4-fold higher C_{max} and an 11.1-fold higher $AUC_{0-\infty}$ when administered as the preformed metabolite compared to when it was administered as the parent **47** (**47M1** C_{max} = 0.54 ± 0.07 μM and **47M1** $AUC_{0-\infty}$ = 8.4 ± 0.4 μM.h). The favourable PK profile of **47M1** combined with its high *in vitro Pf*3D7 potency suggests that **47M1** could demonstrate favourable *in vivo* antimalarial activity.

Table 3.10. Non-compartmental PK parameters of **47M1** following single oral and IV administrations of 20 and 5 mg/kg, respectively of **47M1** to healthy mice

PK parameter[a]	47M1	
	Oral[b]	IV[c]
C_{max} (μM)	9.4 ± 0.5	-
T_{max} (h)	1.7 ± 0.8	-
$T_{1/2}$ (h)	7 ± 1	7.4 ± 0.2
Cl (ml/min/kg)	-	0.15 ± 0.02
V_d (l/kg)	-	0.10 ± 0.02
$AUC_{0-\infty}$ (μM.h)	93 ± 9	62 ± 8
F (%)	42.0	-

[a]Values reported as the mean ± SEM. [b]*n* = 3. [c]*n* = 2 (animal lost during the anaesthesia procedure).

3.3.10. *In vitro-in vivo* absorption, distribution, metabolism, and elimination relationship

The *in vitro* ADME data of the PDBQ parents and major metabolites, as discussed in **Section 3.1.3**, was analysed in conjunction with the previously-presented *in vivo* PK data to determine whether the *in vivo-in vitro* ADME results hold any correlation. In general, a disconnect was observed between the high *in vitro* metabolic Cl_{int} and the low *in vivo* Cl of the parent compounds. The *in vitro* metabolic Cl_{int} is evaluated in the absence of plasma proteins, whereas the *in vivo* Cl takes into account PPB, therefore, the observed low Cl could likely be as a result of PPB or compound accumulation within the murine blood cell, which possibly delayed the elimination of the compound.

The metabolites generally displayed similarly low rates of *in vitro* metabolic Cl_{int} and *in vivo* Cl; however, the low Cl of the metabolites does not correlate with their moderate to low F. Furthermore, the *in vitro* kinetic solubility and permeability data suggests that the metabolites should display moderate to high absorption, however, they displayed moderate to low oral exposure. More insight into the effect of pH on the equilibrium solubility across the GIT is needed to fully understand the oral absorption of the metabolites.

3.3.11. Lead candidate selection

As discussed in **Section 3.1.5**, the deciding PK factors for compound progression were determined by a favourable C_{max}, $AUC_{0\text{-}\infty}$, and the duration in which the systemic concentration remained above the respective *in vitro* *Pf*3D7 IC_{50}. In general, the oral exposure of the preformed metabolites surpassed the combined oral exposure of the parents and formed metabolites. This suggests that the exposure of the PDBQ pharmacophore after parent compound administration might not be as effective as its exposure after administration of the preformed metabolite. Furthermore, the C_{max} values of the preformed metabolites substantially exceeded those of the parent and formed metabolites. Together these observations signify that the administration of the parent compound should not be used as a strategy to deliver the active metabolites. Additionally, the metabolites exhibited greater *in vitro* antimalarial potency than the parents, as shown in **Chapter I, Table 1.1**, which further supports direct administration of the preformed metabolite over the parent compound.

All preformed metabolites displayed a low V_d, which is advantageous since the PDBQ target site is within the vascular system. All preformed metabolites displayed slow Cl which can contribute towards sustained antimalarial exposure. Preformed **43M1** and **47M1** attained relatively high C_{max} values of 8 ± 1 and 9.4 ± 0.5 μM, respectively. Furthermore, preformed **43M1** and **47M1** exhibited the highest $AUC_{0-\infty}$ values of 62 ± 3 and 93 ± 9 μM.h, respectively, and displayed the highest F of approximately 42% compared to the other preformed metabolites. The circulating concentrations of **43M1** and **47M1** were well above their respective *Pf*3D7 IC_{50} values for up to 24 h post-oral administration, which could translate to sustained and effective antimalarial activity. In line with these PK considerations and the *in vitro* activity and selectivity profiles, preformed **43M1** and **47M1** were chosen as lead candidates to be investigated for their antimalarial efficacy in the *P. falciparum*-infected humanised murine model.

3.4. CONCLUSION

An extensive investigation into the PK of the PDBQ parent compounds and active metabolites was performed in a healthy murine model. The findings from these PK studies and the *in vitro* characterisation data were used to determine which compounds were most likely to display *in vivo* antimalarial efficacy. To this end, based on their favourable PK profiles and high *in vitro* antimalarial potency, **43M1** and **47M1** were chosen as lead candidates to be further evaluated for their efficacy in a *P. falciparum*-infected humanised murine model.

CHAPTER IV

IN VIVO PHARMACOKINETICS AND PHARMACODYNAMICS IN A MALARIA-INFECTED MURINE MODEL

4.1. INTRODUCTION

4.1.1. Chapter aim

This chapter investigates the *in vivo* antimalarial efficacy, potency, and PK/PD relationship of the lead candidate PDBQ compounds, **43M1** and **47M1**, in a *P. falciparum*-infected humanised murine model.

4.1.2. A brief introduction to pharmacodynamics

PK describes the time course of drug concentration and how it differs with varying dose, whereas PD describes the physiological effect of the drug on the body. PK/PD analysis aims to define the relationship between dose, or concentration, and the resulting response, which provides insights into drug efficacy and can aid in rational dose prediction for translational studies. PK/PD is based on the inherent assumption that the intensity of a pharmacological response is dependent on the concentration of the drug at its site of action; where higher drug concentrations elicit greater responses until the maximum therapeutic effect is reached[118,140,147,148].

The PK parameters which govern *in vivo* antimalarial efficacy are the maximum concentration, the overall exposure, and the duration in which the peripheral drug concentration remains above the defined minimum therapeutic concentration or threshold concentration[142,143,144]. When the circulating drug concentration falls below the therapeutic range, the rate of parasiticidal activity and antimalarial efficacy will decrease. By establishing the PK/PD relationships which define the maximal response, the dose can be optimised to maintain blood levels above the threshold concentration and, thereby, promote a sustained duration of active exposure[149].

The PD endpoint is distinguished by the suppressive effect of a drug on parasite proliferation in peripheral blood. This can be achieved by inhibiting parasite development and function at various stages of the lifecycle to ultimately prevent erythrocyte reinvasion[150]. Antimalarial PD is quantified by the reduction in parasitaemia of the treatment group relative to the untreated group, and this PD metric measures drug efficacy. The dose-effect relationship is determined using multiple dose levels, and characterises the effective dose required to produce 90% of the maximal parasiticidal response (ED_{90}), which provides a measure of drug potency. Additionally, the maximal concentration and the overall exposure required to produce the effect at the ED_{90} can be determined to further describe the concentration-effect relationship[151].

4.1.3. The *Plasmodium falciparum*-infected humanised murine model

Preclinical animal models are used to evaluate the *in vivo* efficacy of a compound and elucidate the PK/PD relationship within a system which integrates *in vivo* drug disposition with *in vivo* drug activity. Within the scope of malaria, early *in vivo* efficacy studies are primarily performed in murine species which are infected with host-specific forms of *Plasmodium* such as *P. berghei* and *P. yoelli*. Given the host specificity of *Plasmodium*, the clinically relevant species, *P. falciparum*, is unable to survive in non-primate models, and, therefore, rodent species of malaria are used as surrogates to study the efficacy against human malaria infection. However, due to variations in drug response and disease pathology, including differences in growth kinetics between *Plasmodium* species, antimalarial activity against the rodent forms of malaria cannot always be directly translated to the activity against the human infectious forms of malaria[152,153]. Consequently, humanised murine models have been developed which support infection with *P. falciparum* and, therefore, provide a more accurate evaluation of the *in vivo* antimalarial activity against human infection.

Humanised mice are immunocompromised, with defects in their innate and adaptive immunity, which enables them to support engraftment of functional human cells and tissues. Nonobese diabetic (NOD)/severe combined immunodeficiency (*scid*) mice, which harbour a knockout mutation on the γ-chain of the interleukin-2 receptor (IL-2Rγ^{null}), are used to study human malaria. The NOD/*scid* IL-2Rγ^{null} or NSG mouse displays functional defects in the thymus cells and bone marrow cells, and exhibit deficiencies in natural killer cell activity, in addition to other innate immune response defects. NSG mice are engrafted with human erythrocytes which permit the infection, asexual blood-stage development, and replication of *P. falciparum*[154,155,156]. This experimental animal model provides a valuable tool for drug discovery as *in vivo* antimalarial activity can now be directly studied against a *P. falciparum* infection.

A *P. falciparum*-infected NSG murine model was developed by Jiménez-Díaz *et al.* to evaluate the efficacy of preclinical compounds against asexual intraerythrocytic stages of human malaria infection; and this experimental model was employed to determine the antimalarial efficacy and PK/PD relationship of the lead PDBQ candidates[157]. Briefly, NSG mice are engrafted through intraperitoneal (IP) injection with human erythrocytes for at least 10 days prior to infection. The engrafted cells migrate across the peritoneum into the vascular system presumably through lymphatic drainage. Although NSG mice are immunodeficient, they still possess residual immune function which allows them to selectively eliminate the engrafted cells; therefore, daily IP supplementation with human erythrocytes is required to maintain chimerism and sustain the *P. falciparum* infection. Mice are only infected once adequate chimerism has been achieved, which is exhibited by a human erythrocyte population that is greater than the murine erythrocyte population. On day 0, mice are intravenously infected with a preadapted CQS strain of *P. falciparum* *Pf*3D7$^{0087/N9}$, which was specifically selected for its ability to produce reproducible and persistent infections in engrafted NSG mice. The infection is then left to establish for 3 days before the treatment regimen can commence. Following the conclusion of treatment, the suppressive effect of the test compound can be determined by comparing the parasitaemia of the treatment group to an untreated group which is expected to display normal parasite proliferation. The percentage engraftment and degree of parasite burden in peripheral blood samples are measured using flow cytometry methods[157,158].

Flow cytometry is a technique which measures and analyses the properties of single-celled particles suspended in liquid as they travel through a narrow beam of light. Relative cell size, complexity, and fluorescence intensity are some of the characteristics that can be detected with flow cytometry. A flow cytometry system is composed of three components, the fluidics system which transports cells to the optics system for analysis; the optics system which consists of the light source and the excitation and collection optics; and the electronic system which converts incident light signals to electronic signals. In summary, as a cell passes through the laser, it deflects the incident light. Incident laser light which strikes the cell surface continues to travel in the same forward direction and is referred to as forward-scattered light (FSC). When the incident laser light strikes granular intracellular structures, the light refracts and reflects, and this is termed side-scattered light (SSC). FSC gives a measure of cell size, whereas SSC represents the internal complexity of the cell.

Additionally, fluorescent signals from the cell can be collected by detecting the specific emission spectrum of the fluorochrome after laser excitation at the appropriate wavelength. The collected light signals are detected and illustrated on a dot plot where each dot represents a single cell and the relative position on the XY plane is determined by the intensities of the FSC, SSC, or fluorescence. Cell populations can, therefore, be differentiated based on their characteristic light scattering and fluorescent properties[159,160].

As described by Jiménez-Díaz *et al.*, the *P. falciparum*-infected NSG murine model uses flow cytometry techniques to determine the human erythrocyte engraftment and parasitaemia levels in murine peripheral blood[161]. This is achieved by first measuring the total erythrocyte population using its characteristic FSC and SSC, and then, subsequently analysing the murine erythrocyte and parasitised human erythrocyte (phE) subpopulations through their distinct fluorescent signals. The murine erythrocyte subpopulation is distinguished from human erythrocytes using a TER-119 antimouse erythrocyte monoclonal antibody (mAb) which is conjugated to phycoerythrin (PE). The TER-119 mAb reacts with an antigen specifically present on the surface of murine erythrocytes. To allow detection of TER-119 binding, the mAb is labelled with a PE fluorochrome. The emission spectrum of PE is measured on the flow cytometer using the PE or fluorescence (FL-) 2 detector on a Becton Dickinson (BD) flow cytometer[162]. The relative percentage of human erythrocytes is back-calculated using the measured subpopulation of murine erythrocytes and the total erythrocyte population. phE are detected with a nucleic acid dye, SYTO-16, which emits a green fluorescence when bound to nucleic acid. The emission spectrum of STYO 16 is measured with the fluorescein (FITC) or FL1 detector on the BD flow cytometer. Each positive signal that is detected in the FITC channel corresponds to a parasitised cell; therefore, the parasitaemia can be directly determined as a percentage of the total erythrocyte population which receives a positive signal for SYTO-16. The emission spectra of PE and SYTO-16 overlap in the PE and FITC channels, respectively, which results in a false increase in the fluorescence signal. Colour compensation can be used to correct for this by subtracting the overlapping signal of PE in the FITC channel and vice versa[161].

Since nucleic acid expression varies at different stages of the parasite's lifecycle, the intensity of the SYTO-16 signal can be used as a marker to identify the approximate morphological stage of the parasite. Ring-phase parasites have the lowest nucleic acid content with deoxyribonucleic acid (DNA) only. During the early trophozoite stage, DNA replication commences where parasites begin to synthesise ribonucleic acid (RNA); this results in an accumulation of nucleic acid as the parasite matures to the late trophozoite stage and reaches a peak at the schizont stage[163,164,165]. This suggests that the intensity of the SYTO-16 fluorescence signal will progressively increase as the parasite develops from the ring phase to the schizont phase. **Figure 4.1** presents an illustrative flow cytometry dot plot of an unsynchronised population of *P. falciparum*-infected humanised murine whole blood from an NSG mouse. The phE cells have been stained with SYTO-16, and the murine erythrocyte subpopulation has been marked with TER-119-PE mAb. The exact morphological stages of the parasites cannot be explicitly delineated, and, therefore, the theoretical subpopulations of the parasite phases have been defined based on their relative nucleic acid levels as determined by the corresponding SYTO-16 fluorescence intensity[161,166].

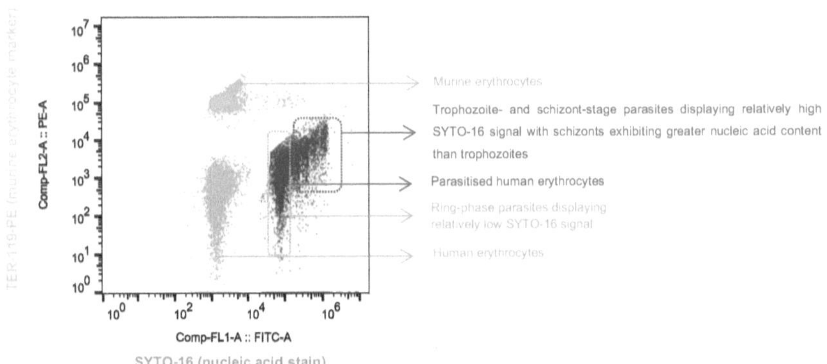

Figure 4.1. Flow cytometry dot plot of *P. falciparum*-infected humanised murine blood from an NSG mouse. The murine erythrocytes were marked with TER-119-PE mAb and the parasites were stained with SYTO-16 nucleic acid dye. The theoretical morphological stages of the parasites are distinguished based on the relative nucleic acid content and the corresponding SYTO-16 fluorescence intensity.

4.1.4. Pharmacokinetic and pharmacodynamic study design in a malaria-infected murine model

This proof of concept study was designed to evaluate the PK/PD of the lead PDBQ candidates, **43M1** and **47M1**, in a *P. falciparum*-infected humanised murine model. The *in vivo* antimalarial activity of **43M1** and **47M1** was determined against asexual intraerythrocytic parasites as the PDBQ compounds are expected to act during this phase of the parasite lifecycle when haemoglobin metabolism is occurring[77]. As presented in **Chapter III**, **43M1** and **47M1** were chosen as lead candidates from the PDBQ series of compounds; based on their relatively high *in vitro* antiplasmodial potency and selectivity, as shown in **Chapter I**, **Table 1.1**, and their favourable *in vivo* oral PK as determined in a healthy murine model.

The efficacy experiments were performed using the Peters' four-day challenge test, which evaluates the changes in parasitaemia after four consecutive daily oral administrations of the test compound[167]. Additionally, to monitor the performance of the experimental procedure, each study included a negative or untreated control group and a positive reference control group. The parasitaemia was measured every 24 h from the first administration to 24 h after the last administration. Since mice were inoculated with an asynchronous infection, the efficacy endpoint encompassed at least 2 complete asexual intraerythrocytic lifecycles of 48 h, from the ring phase to the merozoite phase when reinvasion occurs. The therapeutic activity was determined by comparing the degree of parasite suppression or parasite proliferation of the treatment group to the untreated control group 24 h after the last oral administration.

In order to establish the dose-response relationship of **43M1** and **47M1**, a series of 5 doses were administered to cover a wide range from 0.2–40 mg/kg. Compound potency was evaluated by the ED_{90} value, which measured the dose that resulted in a 90% reduction in parasitaemia with respect to the untreated control group 24 h after the last oral administration. To correlate the drug exposure to the parasiticidal activity, the PK of each test compound was determined after single oral administrations of each dose. The PK/PD parameters that were determined were the maximum concentration required to produce 90% of the maximal parasiticidal response ($C_{maxED90}$) and the oral exposure required to produce 90% of the maximal parasiticidal response (AUC_{ED90}).

Lastly, in order to illustrate and evaluate the duration of effective antimalarial activity, a minimum therapeutic concentration was determined using each compound's *in vitro* activity against *Pf*3D7, as displayed in **Chapter I, Table 1.1**. Generally, the threshold concentration is set to be twice the inhibitory concentration that produces 99% of the maximal parasiticidal response (IC_{99}). However, the IC_{99} values could not be determined from the *in vitro* dose-response curves obtained for **43M1** and **47M1** against *Pf*3D7; therefore, it was proposed that the defined theoretical minimal therapeutic concentration to be used in this study should be conservatively set at four times each compound's respective *in vitro* *Pf*3D7 IC_{50} value[144,149].

4.2. METHODS

4.2.1. Ethics statement

The *in vivo* PK and antimalarial efficacy evaluations were performed in immunocompromised NSG mice at the Drug Discovery and Development Centre (H3D), Division of Clinical Pharmacology, UCT. Ethical approval was granted before commencement of these studies by the Animal Ethics Committee of the FHS, UCT. The ethics reference number is 017/025.

4.2.2. Animal housing

Efficacy experiments were performed in 6–10 week old, male NOD/*scid* IL-2Rγ^{null} mice, weighing between 25–35 g. Mice were housed and maintained throughout the experimental procedure in a sterile environment, and water and food were supplied *ad libitum.* The mice were monitored daily for distress and discomfort during the engraftment procedure and then twice a day after infection with *P. falciparum.* Animal husbandry and experimental procedures were followed in accordance with the guidelines of the FHS Animal Ethics Committee, UCT.

4.2.3. Materials and instrumentation

43M1 and **47M1** were upscaled for the efficacy experiments at the Department of Chemistry, UCT. Both compounds showed HPLC-MS purity > 98%. The materials and instrumentation used for the HPLC-MS/MS PK analysis, and those used to prepare the oral dosing vehicle are described in **Chapter II**, **Section 2.2.1** and **Section 2.2.2**. Additional materials and instrumentation used for the *in vivo* antimalarial efficacy evaluations in NSG mice are described here and in **Table 4.1**. Human whole blood was obtained from the blood bank at Groote Schuur Hospital, Cape Town. NSG mice were originally obtained from the Jackson Laboratory (Jackson Laboratory, Maine, US) and were subsequently bred at the UCT Research Animal Facility, Cape Town. *P. falciparum Pf*3D7$^{0087/N9}$ parasites were obtained from GlaxoSmithKline Tres Cantos Medicines Development Campus, Madrid, Spain. Human erythrocyte engraftment and parasitaemia measurements were determined using a BD Accuri C6 Plus flow cytometer (BD, New Jersey, US) and data acquisition was performed using BD CSampler Plus software version 1.0.23.1 (BD, New Jersey, US).

Table 4.1. List of materials used for the *in vivo* efficacy evaluation in *P. falciparum*-infected NSG mice and the suppliers from which they were purchased

Material	Supplier
CQ diphosphate	Sigma-Aldrich (Merck, Missouri, US)
Glutaraldehyde	Sigma-Aldrich
Heat inactivated AB+ human serum	Sigma-Aldrich
Hypoxanthine	Sigma-Aldrich
Phosphate buffered saline (PBS)	Gibco (Thermo Fisher Scientific, Massachusetts, US)
RPMI-1640 medium	Gibco
SYTO-16	Invitrogen (Thermo Fisher Scientific, Massachusetts, US)
TER-119-PE mAb	BioLegend (BioLegend, California, US)
Trucount beads	BD (BD, New Jersey, US)

4.2.4. Engraftment and infection in humanised mice

The *in vivo* efficacy studies conducted in the *P. falciparum*-infected humanised murine model were performed using the methods described by Jiménez-Díaz *et al.*[157] For at least 10 days prior to the day of *P. falciparum* infection, NSG mice were engrafted daily with prepared human erythrocytes through IP injection. Briefly, washed human erythrocytes were prepared to a 50% haematocrit in a solution of RPMI 1640, 25% (v/v) decomplemented human serum, and 3.1 mM hypoxanthine. The human erythrocyte suspension was then warmed to 37°C before 1 ml of the solution was injected intraperitoneally into the mouse. Daily engraftments continued during compound administration to maintain adequate chimerism in the peripheral blood. The uptake of the engraftment was routinely monitored by measuring the percentage of human erythrocytes relative to the total erythrocyte population[157,158]. The peripheral human erythrocyte and parasitaemia levels were concurrently measured using the flow cytometry method described by Jiménez-Díaz *et al.*[161] In summary, blood samples were collected from each experimental mouse via tail vein bleeding into lithium heparin tubes. Two microlitre blood aliquots were then incubated for 20 min, in the dark at ambient temperature, with 100 µl 5% (v/v) TER-119-PE mAb and

0.5% (v/v) SYTO-16 in PBS. Samples were fixed with 10 µl 0.25% (v/v) glutaraldehyde in PBS and finally diluted tenfold with PBS before flow cytometry analysis[161].

The flow cytometry analysis was performed using a BD Accuri C6 Plus flow cytometer, and data acquisition was performed using BD CSampler Plus software version 1.0.23.1. The acquisition method was set to collect 1 million cell events in the total erythrocyte population. FSC and SSC were set to detect the total erythrocyte population, and the fluorescence of SYTO-16 and TER-119-PE mAb in the erythrocyte population were detected in the FITC and PE channels, respectively. Colour compensation was performed in the FITC and PE channels. As determined by the sensitivity of the flow cytometer, the lower limit of parasitaemia detection was 0.01%[161].

Experimental mice were infected with *P. falciparum* only once the percentage engraftment of human erythrocytes was ≥ 50% of the total erythrocyte population. On the day of infection, day 0, mice were intravenously injected in the tail vein with 2 x 10^7 asynchronous *P. falciparum Pf*3D7$^{0087/N9}$ parasites. The parasites were obtained from the NSG donor mice, which were harbouring *Pf*3D7$^{0087/N9}$ infected human erythrocytes. In order to determine the volume of blood which corresponded to 2 x 10^7 parasites, the concentration of phE was measured using calibrated fluorescent BD Trucount beads, which are detected by flow cytometry. Briefly, a known number and concentration of fluorescent Trucount beads were added to each donor mouse peripheral blood sample, which were stained with SYTO-16 and TER-119-PE mAb, as described above. The number of acquired bead events correlated to the volume of the sample that was used to determine the total erythrocyte cell count. Therefore, the actual concentration of erythrocytes was determined by dividing the number of erythrocyte events by the number of bead events and then multiplying that by the known concentration of beads. Subsequently, the concentration of phE was determined by comparing the parasitaemia to the calculated concentration of erythrocytes. Once inoculated, the mice were left for 3 days to allow the infection to establish before commencement of compound administration[157,161].

4.2.5. Compound administration and sampling

The antimalarial efficacies of **43M1** and **47M1** were assessed using the four-day suppressive test as described by Peters[167]. The first day of treatment corresponded to day 3, which was three days after the experimental mice were infected. Test compounds and controls were administered by oral gavage once a day for 4 consecutive days from day 3 to 6. The oral dosing groups for **43M1** and **47M1** were 0.2, 2, 10, 20, and 40 mg/kg/day. Additionally, the negative control group was orally administered with the oral dosing vehicle, which was free of the test compound; and the positive control group was orally administered with 20 mg/kg/day of CQ. Mice were randomly assigned to each treatment group ($n = 2$). The test compounds were administered in the oral dosing vehicle consisting of 0.5% (w/v) HPMC in H_2O with 0.2% (v/v) Tween80®, which was sterile filtered through a 0.22 µm membrane before compound preparation. First, the 40 mg/kg dose was prepared, this was then serially diluted with the sterile filtered dosing vehicle to prepare the administrations for the lower dosage groups. The test compound formulations were freshly prepared each day before administration on days 3, 4, 5, and 6 post-infection. The negative control group was prepared with 0.22 µm sterile-filtered 0.5% (w/v) HPMC in H_2O with 0.2% (v/v) Tween80®, and the 20 mg/kg CQ formulation was prepared in sterile PBS.

The whole blood samples, used to assess the PK and efficacy, were collected via tail vein bleeding into lithium heparin tubes. The PK samples were collected for each test compound dosing group at 0.5, 1, 3, 5, 7, and 24 h after the first administration on day 3. PK samples were temporarily stored on ice before being transferred to -80°C for storage, until the HPLC-MS/MS analysis. Efficacy blood samples were collected for all dosing groups, before compound administration, on days 3, 4, 5, 6, and 7. These samples were processed immediately after collection to determine the parasitaemia and the percentage engraftment, as described in **Section 4.2.4**.

4.2.6. Pharmacodynamic analysis

The antimalarial activity was monitored by measuring the changes in peripheral blood parasitaemia from days 3–7. Parasitaemia values were determined on BD CSampler Plus software version 1.0.23.1, and flow cytometry dot plots were generated using FlowJo software version 10.6.1 (BD, New Jersey, US). The percentage reduction in parasitaemia was determined by comparing the parasitaemia of the treatment group to the parasitaemia of the untreated group on day 7 post-infection. The ED_{90} was calculated to evaluate the dose-effect relationship. In GraphPad Prism software version 4, a sigmoidal dose-response curve was fitted to the log_{10}(dose) and the corresponding mean log_{10}(% parasitaemia) relative to the negative control on day 7. The ED_{90} value was then interpolated from the generated curve. Graphical representations and statistical analyses were performed in GraphPad Prism software version 4. The parasitaemia values are displayed as the mean ± SEM.

4.2.7. Pharmacokinetic analysis

Quantification of **43M1** and **47M1** in humanised murine whole blood was performed according to the relevant bioanalytical procedure as described in **Section 2.3.2**. Briefly, PK study samples and matrix-matched calibration standard and QC samples were removed from -80°C storage and left to thaw on ice. Calibration standard and QC samples were analysed in duplicate. Analytes were extracted using protein precipitation with ice-cold 0.1% (v/v) NH_4OH in ACN spiked with the ISTD **126**. Samples were vortexed for 1 min and then centrifuged at 5590 x *g* for 5 min. The resulting supernatant was then diluted twofold with 0.1% (v/v) NH_4OH in H_2O. All samples were submitted for HPLC-MS/MS analysis using an Agilent 1260 Infinity II HPLC system (Agilent Technologies, California, US) coupled to a SCIEX API 5500 (SCIEX, Toronto, Canada). The unknown analyte concentrations in the experimental PK samples were determined using Analyst software version 1.6.3 (SCIEX, Toronto, Canada).

Concentration-time profiles and the $C_{maxED90}$ and AUC_{ED90} values were determined in GraphPad Prism software version 4. In addition to the concentration-time profile, a log_{10}(concentration)-time profile was plotted against each compound's respective threshold concentration, which was set at 4 times their *in vitro Pf*3D7 IC_{50}, as displayed in **Chapter I, Table 1.1**. The PK parameters, C_{max}, T_{max}, and the area under the concentration-time curve from time 0–24 h ($AUC_{0\text{-}24}$), were determined using NCA in PK Solver software, as described in **Section 3.2.6**[145]. The PK parameters are presented as the mean ± SEM. The mean $log_{10}(C_{max})$ or mean $log_{10}(AUC_{0\text{-}24})$ values obtained for each dosing group were fitted with a sigmoidal dose-response curve to the corresponding mean log_{10}(% parasitaemia) relative to the negative control on day 7. The $C_{maxED90}$ and AUC_{ED90} values were then interpolated from the generated curves. Additionally, the dose-normalised C_{max} and $AUC_{0\text{-}24}$ values were determined by dividing each derived PK parameter value by their respective dose.

The presented compound concentration and PK data represent the total concentration as values were not corrected for PPB, compound accumulation within the erythrocyte, and compound accumulation within the parasite[158,168].

4.3. RESULTS AND DISCUSSION

4.3.1. Review of the *in vivo* efficacy experimental procedure

The *in vivo* efficacy and PK measurements for **43M1** and **47M1** in *P. falciparum*-infected NSG mice were performed over two independent studies. The presented parasitaemia levels of the untreated and CQ control groups were averaged using the data obtained from both studies. **43M1** was evaluated in the first study; but, during treatment between days 4–7, the peripheral blood chimerism fell below 50% for several mice, which resulted in unproductive infections. The unsustained engraftment is hypothesised to be due to the experimental procedure rather than as a result of any *in vivo* physiological interactions of the compound. The mice which exhibited unreliable infections were excluded from both the efficacy and PK analyses. The first study produced reliable results for the 0.2, 10, and 20 mg/kg groups; but, only one replicate was obtained for each dosing group. Both mice in the 2 and 40 mg/kg dosing groups did not maintain their engraftment to day 7. In order to obtain strong data and an accurate ED_{90} value, selected dosing groups of **43M1** were administered again in the second study, namely the 2 mg/kg group (n = 2) and the 10 and 20 mg/kg groups (n = 1 for each dose level). Since there was a limited number of mice in the second study, all dosing groups of **43M1** could not be retested. The maximal effect of **43M1** was hypothesised to occur at 20 mg/kg; therefore, the 40 mg/kg group was excluded. Additionally, the usable result of the 0.2 mg/kg group of **43M1** revealed this dose to be ineffective, as displayed by an increase in parasitaemia that was comparable to the negative control group (data not shown); therefore, this treatment group was also not included in the second study. There were no difficulties encountered with the engraftment during the second study, and all results for **47M1** were included in the PK/PD analysis.

Importantly, for both **43M1** and **47M1**, mice did not display signs of toxicity or distress in all of the dosing groups, including the highest group of 40 mg/kg, which was well tolerated after the quadruple dosing regimen.

4.3.2. Review of the bioanalytical method performance

The HPLC-MS/MS bioanalytical methods used for the quantification of **43M1** or **47M1** in humanised murine whole blood, as described in **Section 2.3.2**, performed well during the PK sample analysis, and fulfilled the criteria that was required to accept the analytical batch, as discussed in **Chapter II, Section 2.1.3.7**. The PK samples for each analyte were analysed in two separate batches. In general, there were no problems encountered with chromatography, sensitivity, selectivity, and carryover. Quadratic regression with a 1/x weighting (r > 0.99) was used to fit the calibration curves for both analytes, which covered the concentration range from 2–4000 ng/ml. Each PK batch of **43M1** and **47M1** displayed acceptable assay accuracy and precision for the calibration standard and QC samples[98]. The determined concentrations of **43M1** and **47M1** in the NSG mice were lower than the expected concentrations, which were determined using the concentration data that was obtained from the PK experiments in healthy C57BL/6 mice, as presented in **Chapter III**. For this reason, the calibration curves which covered the higher quantification range, between 75–8000 ng/ml for **43M1** and 75–10000 ng/ml for **47M1**, were not used for the quantitative analysis. A summary of the representative chromatograms, calibration curves, and statistical data for each PK batch of **43M1** and **47M1** is presented in **Appendix B**. Of note, several experimental PK samples were unable to be accurately aliquoted during sample preparation as the whole blood had clotted. This could be due to insufficient mixing of the whole blood with the lithium heparin anticoagulant during sample collection, or possibly as a result of unknown physiological factors. These samples were excluded from the PK analysis and are denoted by no experimental sample in the calculated PK concentration tables presented in **Appendix B**.

4.3.3. Pharmacokinetics and pharmacodynamics of 43M1

Figure 4.2 displays the whole blood concentrations of **43M1** following single oral administrations of 2, 10, and 20 mg/kg of **43M1** to *P. falciparum*-infected NSG mice. In the 2 mg/kg group, the circulating concentration of **43M1** did not significantly exceed the threshold concentration of 0.064 μM for 24 h post-administration, as shown in **Figure 4.2.B**. These suboptimal concentration levels could curtail effective therapeutic activity. In the 10 mg/kg group, the circulating concentration of **43M1** fell below the threshold concentration at approximately 20 h post-administration, which could potentially translate to limited antimalarial efficacy. Lastly, for the 20 mg/kg group, **43M1** maintained circulating concentrations above the minimum therapeutic concentration for 24 h post-administration. Additionally, the concentration of **43M1** at 24 h was approximately 1.4-fold higher than the threshold concentration. Therefore, this sustained exposure of **43M1** could permit favourable antimalarial activity.

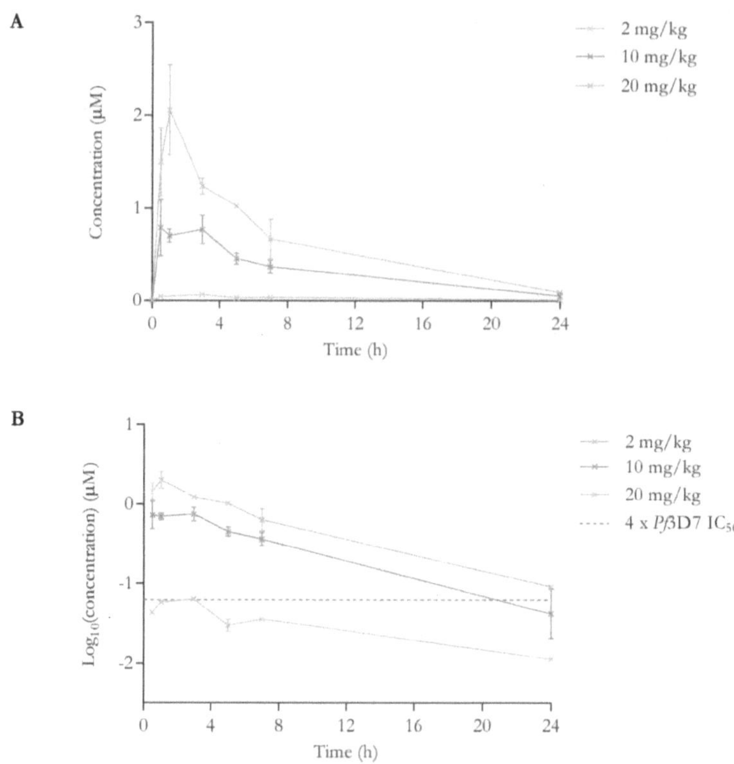

Figure 4.2. Mean (SEM) humanised murine whole blood **A** concentration-time profile and **B** $\log_{10}$(concentration)-time profile against the minimum *in vitro* therapeutic concentration of **43M1** following single oral administrations of 2, 10, and 20 mg/kg of **43M1** to *P. falciparum*-infected NSG mice ($n = 2$).

Figure 4.3 presents the changes in parasitaemia after four consecutive daily oral administrations of 2, 10, and 20 mg/kg of **43M1** to *P. falciparum*-infected NSG mice. The 2 mg/kg dose group was entirely ineffective at suppressing parasite proliferation as displayed by the increase in parasitaemia from day 3 to 7, which was comparable to the untreated group. This could most likely be attributed to the insufficient exposure of **43M1**, as the daily circulating concentration of **43M1** did not surpass its minimum therapeutic concentration, as shown in **Figure 4.2.B**. The 10 mg/kg group displayed a parasite clearance of 75% relative to the untreated group on day 7. The comparatively poor efficacy of the 10 mg/kg dose group could be as a result of the limited exposure of **43M1** as the daily circulating levels of **43M1** fell below the minimum therapeutic concentration at 20 h post-administration, as shown in **Figure 4.2.B**. Lastly, in the 20 mg/kg group, the daily circulating concentration of **43M1** remained above the threshold concentration for 24 h post-administration. This translated to a favourable 98% reduction in parasitaemia relative to the untreated group on day 7. The 20 mg/kg CQ group displayed a reduction in parasitaemia of 99% relative to the untreated group on day 7 which is comparable to the 20 mg/kg group of **43M1**. In general, **43M1** displayed a dose-dependent relationship with the reduction in parasitaemia.

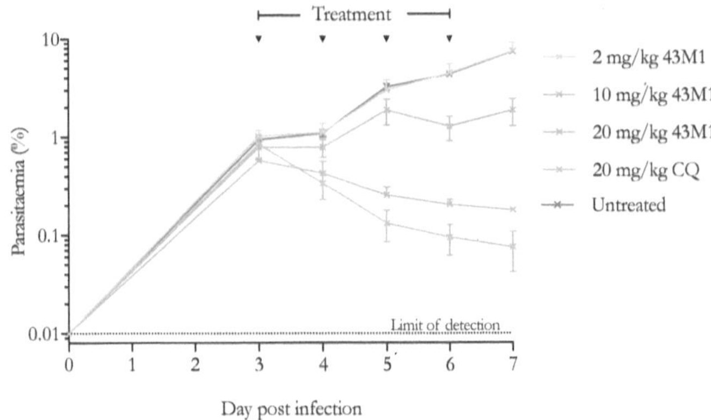

Figure 4.3. Mean (SEM) percent changes in parasitaemia of *P. falciparum* infected in NSG mice following 4 consecutive daily oral administrations of various doses of either **43M1**, CQ, or the oral vehicle only ($n = 2$ per **43M1** dose group and $n = 4$ for the CQ and untreated control groups).

Table 4.2 displays a summary of the PK parameters of **43M1** following single oral administrations of 2, 10, and 20 mg/kg of **43M1** to *P. falciparum*-infected NSG mice. The apparent C_{max} values determined were 0.064 ± 0.002, 1.01 ± 0.08, and 2.1 ± 0.5 μM after administration of 2, 10, and 20 mg/kg of **43M1**, respectively. The T_{max} values ranged from 1 to 3 h, and no pronounced trends were observed with the increase in dose and the rate of oral absorption. The 20 mg/kg group displayed the highest oral exposure of 15 ± 3 μM.h followed by the 10 mg/kg group and then the 2 mg/kg group which displayed AUC_{0-24} values of 7.7 ± 0.2 and 0.714 ± 0.005 μM.h, respectively. The dose-normalised C_{max} and AUC_{0-24} values were approximately proportional at 10 and 20 mg/kg, which suggests that the clearance mechanisms were not saturated at these higher doses. The 2 mg/kg group did not exhibit dose proportionality in C_{max} and AUC_{0-24}, which could possibly be attributed to its lower extent of systemic absorption due to the fast metabolism of NSG mice[169].

Table 4.2. Non-compartmental PK parameters of **43M1** following single oral administrations of 2, 10, and 20 mg/kg of **43M1** to *P. falciparum*-infected NSG mice

PK parameter[a]	**43M1**		
	2 mg/kg[b]	**10 mg/kg**[b]	**20 mg/kg**[b]
C_{max} (μM)	0.064 ± 0.002	1.01 ± 0.08	2.1 ± 0.5
C_{max} /dose (μM/mg/kg)	0.0321 ± 0.0008	0.101 ± 0.008	0.10 ± 0.02
T_{max} (h)	3	2 ± 1	1
AUC_{0-24}(μM.h)	0.714 ± 0.005	7.7 ± 0.2	15 ± 3
AUC_{0-24}/dose (μM.h/mg/kg)	0.357 ± 0.003	0.77 ± 0.02	0.8 ± 0.1

[a]Values reported as the mean ± SEM. [b]n = 2.

Table 4.3 presents the PK/PD parameters of **43M1** in the *P. falciparum*-infected NSG murine model. Ideally, at least 5 dose levels should be used to determine the ED_{90} and concentration-related ED_{90} values; however, the efficacy of **43M1** was measured only at 2, 10, and 20 mg/kg[170]. Nonetheless, the PK/PD parameters could still be calculated as the 90% reduction in parasitaemia fell between 2 and 10 mg/kg. The excluded dose groups of 0.2 and 40 mg/kg of **43M1** presumably displayed minimal and maximal parasiticidal activity, respectively; therefore, the inclusion of these dose groups are hypothesised to not significantly affect the ED_{90} value. Additionally, all dose-response curves displayed goodness of fit values ≥ 0.982, as shown in **Appendix B, Figure B.27**. **43M1** displayed an ED_{90} of 12 mg/kg and corresponding $C_{maxED90}$ and AUC_{ED90} values of 0.81 μM and 6.2 μM.h, respectively.

Table 4.3. PK/PD parameters of **43M1** in a *P. falciparum*-infected NSG murine model

ED_{90} (mg/kg)	12
$C_{maxED90}$ (μM)	0.81
AUC_{ED90} (μM.h)	6.2

4.3.4. Pharmacokinetics and pharmacodynamics of 47M1

Figure 4.4 displays the whole blood concentrations of **47M1** following single oral administrations of 2, 10, 20, and 40 mg/kg of **47M1** to *P. falciparum*-infected NSG mice. **47M1** was detected in all dose groups for 24 h post-administration except for the 0.2 mg/kg group, which displayed concentration values below the LLOQ of 2 ng/ml for the entire sampling period. Troughs and subsequent peaks in analyte concentration were observed between 3 and 7 h in the 10, 20, and 40 mg/kg dose groups, which is proposed to be a consequence of enterohepatic circulation. As shown in **Figure 4.4.B**, **47M1** exhibited sustained exposures at all dosages, as displayed by the circulating concentrations of **47M1,** which exceeded the threshold concentration of 0.052 μM for 24 h post-administration. The concentrations of **47M1** were 2.3-, 11.6-, 20.3-, and 61.3-fold higher than its minimum therapeutic concentration at 24 h post-administration of 2, 10, 20, and 40 mg/kg of **47M1,** respectively.

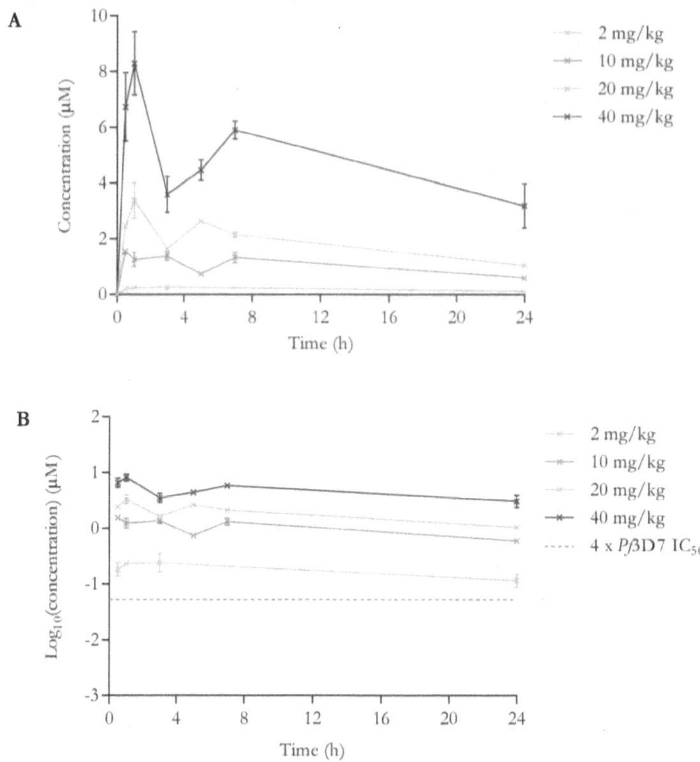

Figure 4.4. Mean (SEM) humanised murine whole blood **A** concentration-time profile and **B** log_{10}(concentration)-time profile against the minimum *in vitro* therapeutic concentration of **47M1** following single oral administrations of 2, 10, 20, and 40 mg/kg of **47M1** to *P. falciparum*-infected NSG mice ($n = 2$).

Figure 4.5 presents the changes in parasitaemia after four consecutive daily oral administrations of 0.2, 2, 10, 20, and 40 mg/kg of **47M1** to *P. falciparum*-infected NSG mice. The 0.2 and 2 mg/kg groups exhibited ineffectual antimalarial activity as displayed by the increase in parasitaemia from day 3 to 7, which was comparable to that of the untreated control group. Although the 2 mg/kg group displayed daily circulating concentrations of **47M1** which exceeded the minimum therapeutic concentration for 24 h post-administration, the levels were insufficient to suppress parasite proliferation. The 10 mg/kg group displayed a 96% reduction in parasitaemia compared to the untreated group on day 7, and the

20 and 40 mg/kg groups both exhibited a 98% parasite clearance compared to the untreated group on day 7, which is similar to that observed for the 20 mg/kg CQ group. The efficacious antimalarial activity of these dosing groups could be attributed to the daily circulating concentrations of **47M1**, which remained at least 10 times above the threshold concentration at 24 h post-administration, as shown in **Figure 4.4.B**. The maximal antimalarial effect of **47M1** was reached at 20 mg/kg since both the 20 and 40 mg/kg groups of **47M1** displayed a comparable 98% reduction in parasitaemia. As observed with **43M1, 47M1** also displayed a dose-dependent relationship with the reduction in parasitaemia.

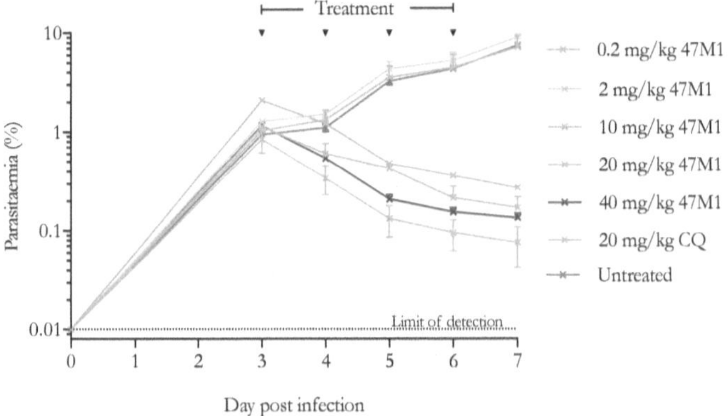

Figure 4.5. Mean (SEM) percent changes in parasitaemia of *P. falciparum* infected in NSG mice following 4 consecutive daily oral administrations of various doses of either **47M1**, CQ, or the oral vehicle only (n = 2 per **47M1** dose group and n = 4 for the CQ and untreated control groups).

Table 4.4 displays a summary of the PK parameters of **47M1** following single oral administrations of 2, 10, 20, and 40 mg/kg of **47M1** to *P. falciparum*-infected NSG mice. The apparent C_{max} reached after administration of 2, 10, 20, and 40 mg/kg of **47M1** were 0.28 ± 0.07, 1.59 ± 0.07, 3.4 ± 0.6, and 8 ± 1 µM, respectively. Additionally, **47M1** exhibited approximate dose-proportional increases in C_{max} across the dosing range from 2–40 mg/kg. The T_{max} values ranged from 0.8 ± 0.3 to 2 ± 1 h which suggests that the higher dose levels of **47M1** did not exhibit any delay in the rate of compound dissolution and oral absorption in the GIT. Similarly to the dose-normalised C_{max} values, the $AUC_{0\text{-}24}$ values of **47M1** were also approximately dose-proportional from 2–40 mg/kg, which suggests that **47M1** did not display saturable clearance at the higher doses. The oral exposures of **47M1** ranged from 5 ± 1 to 113 ± 6 μM.h, as exhibited by the 2 and 40 mg/kg dose groups, respectively.

Table 4.4. Non-compartmental PK parameters of **47M1** following single oral administrations of 2, 10, 20, and 40 mg/kg of **47M1** to *P. falciparum*-infected NSG mice

PK parameter[a]	47M1			
	2 mg/kg[b]	10 mg/kg[b]	20 mg/kg[b]	40 mg/kg[b]
C_{max} (μM)	0.28 ± 0.07	1.59 ± 0.07	3.4 ± 0.6	8 ± 1
C_{max} /dose (μM/mg/kg)	0. 14 ± 0.03	0.159 ± 0.007	0.17 ± 0.03	0.21 ± 0.03
T_{max} (h)	2 ± 1	0.8 ± 0.3	1	1
AUC_{0-24}(μM.h)	5 ± 1	25 ± 3	45 ± 4	113 ± 6
AUC_{0-24}/dose (μM.h/mg/kg)	2.3 ± 0.7	2.5 ± 0.3	2.3 ± 0.2	2.8 ± 0.1

[a]Values reported as the mean ± SEM. [b]n = 2.

Table 4.5 presents the PK/PD parameters of **47M1** in the *P. falciparum*-infected NSG murine mode. **47M1** displayed an ED_{90} of 7.7 mg/kg. The corresponding C_{max} and exposure required to reduce parasite proliferation by 90% were 1.2 μM and 18.6 μM.h, respectively. All dose-response curves used to determine the ED_{90} and concentration-related ED_{90} values displayed goodness of fit values ≥ 0.987, as shown in **Appendix B, Figure B.28**. Given the dose-proportional absorption and clearance kinetics of **47M1**; when treated with the ED_{90} dose of 7.7 mg/kg, the concentration levels of **47M1** are expected to remain above its minimum therapeutic concentration for 24 h post-administration, as shown in **Figure 4.4.B**.

Table 4.5. PK/PD parameters of **47M1** in a *P. falciparum*-infected NSG murine model

ED_{90} (mg/kg)	7.7
$C_{maxED90}$ (µM)	1.2
AUC_{ED90}(µM.h)	18.6

4.3.5. Review of the pharmacokinetics and pharmacodynamics of the lead pyridodibemequine candidates

43M1 and **47M1** were both efficacious in a dose-dependent manner in the *P. falciparum*-infected NSG murine model. The parasiticidal effects observed at each dose level correlate well with the observed peripheral drug concentrations at the site of action. Although **43M1** and **47M1** displayed equipotent *in vitro* antiplasmodial activity against *Pf*3D7, as shown in **Chapter I, Table 1.1**, their *in vivo* antimalarial potency differed where **47M1** displayed a lower ED_{90} of 7.7 mg/kg compared to **43M1** which exhibited an ED_{90} of 12 mg/kg. This disconnect can be attributed to differences in each compound's PK profile as displayed by the C_{max} and $AUC_{0\text{-}24}$ values where **47M1** generally displayed higher oral absorption and exposure compared to **43M1** at the equivalent doses. Furthermore, the higher observed *in vivo* potency of **47M1** can be attributed to the AUC_{ED90} values where **47M1** exhibited a 3.0-fold higher exposure at the ED_{90} compared to **43M1**. The efficacious dose groups of **43M1** (20 mg/kg) and **47M1** (10, 20, and 40 mg/kg) displayed an immediate onset of action within the first 24 h of treatment as observed by the parasitaemia levels which decreased from day 3 to 4. In general, the rate of oral absorption was not prolonged at the higher doses of **43M1** and **47M1**. Additionally, C_{max} and $AUC_{0\text{-}24}$ increased relatively proportionally to the increase in dose between 10 and 20 mg/kg for **43M1** and between 2 and 40 mg/kg for **47M1**, which suggests linear elimination kinetics over the specified dose ranges.

Inconsistent compound exposures were observed between the PK studies in healthy C57BL/6 mice, as presented in **Chapter III**, and those performed here in *P. falciparum*-infected NSG mice. After oral administrations of 20 mg/kg of either **43M1** or **47M1** in 0.5% (w/v) HPMC in H_2O with 0.2% (v/v) Tween80®, the observed analyte concentration in the NSG murine model did not reach as high a level as those displayed in the C57BL/6 murine model, as shown in **Appendix B, Section B.3**. The overall oral exposure of **43M1** was 4.1-fold lower in the NSG model compared to the C57BL/6 model (C57BL/6 $AUC_{0\text{-}24}$ = 62 ± 3 μM.h and NSG $AUC_{0\text{-}24}$ = 15 ± 3 μM.h); and the exposure of **47M1** was 2.1-fold lower in the NSG model compared to the C57BL/6 model (C57BL/6 $AUC_{0\text{-}24}$ = 93 ± 9 μM.h and NSG $AUC_{0\text{-}24}$ = 45 ± 4 μM.h). The lower oral exposure observed in the NSG mice could be attributed to differences in the hepatic metabolic processes between each murine species. It has been previously suggested that NSG mice could exhibit faster metabolism than C57BL/6 mice, which results in higher clearance and therefore lower systemic exposure in NSG mice[169]. Additionally, the disease state could have influenced the PK profiles of **43M1** and **47M1**, however, the PK profile in uninfected NSG mice and the degree of compound accumulation in infected erythrocytes will first need to be determined to elucidate the relationship between the PK in the healthy and infected mice. Lastly, the observed variability in oral exposure between each murine model could be attributed to differences in compound solubility between synthesised batches. **43M1** and **47M1** were upscaled for the experiments in the NSG model; therefore, the administered compound in the C57BL/6 murine model was from a different batch to the compound administered in the NSG murine model. Inconsistencies with the solubility in the dosing vehicle and at physiologically relevant pH environments could have occurred between the different batches, and the possibility of this should be further investigated.

Figure 4.6 displays the representative changes in the *P. falciparum* population in chimeric NSG mice after treatment with 20 mg/kg of either **43M1** or **47M1** compared to an untreated control group. The observed changes in the conceptualised subpopulations of rings, trophozoites, and schizonts are based upon the relative nucleic acid content between each morphological stage and the corresponding relative SYTO-16 fluorescence intensity where schizont-stage parasites display the highest signal in FITC followed by trophozoites, and lastly, ring-stage parasites which exhibit the lowest signal in FITC, as described in **Section 4.1.3** and **Figure 4.1**[161,165,166]. The untreated control group displays the normal progression of infection in the absence of antimalarial therapy. **Figure 4.6.A** shows a relatively unsynchronised population of parasites on day 3; however, the predominant phase does appear to be the ring stage. On day 4, **Figure 4.6.B**, higher SYTO-16 fluorescence signals are observed in the untreated group which corresponds to an increase in parasite nucleic acid levels as a result of the maturation of the day 3 ring-stage parasites to trophozoite- and schizont-stage parasites on day 4. Day 5, **Figure 4.6.C**, exhibits the completion of a 48 h lifecycle where ring-stage parasites predominate once again. Additionally, a significant increase in parasitaemia from day 4 to 5 is observed, which corresponds to erythrocyte reinvasion by merozoites. The parasite population on day 6, **Figure 4.6.D**, shows the maturation of ring-stage parasites to trophozoites and schizonts as indicated by the increase in SYTO-16 fluorescence, which corresponds to the increased DNA and RNA levels in developing trophozoites and schizonts[163]. Lastly, on day 7, **Figure 4.6.E**, subsequent reinfection by schizont rupture is exhibited; as displayed by the increase in the number of infected human erythrocytes. Similar to the untreated group, mice treated with **43M1** or **47M1** displayed predominately ring-stage parasites on day 3, as shown in **Figure 4.6.F** and **K**, respectively. As shown in **Figure 4.6.G** and **L**, the parasitaemia of the treatment groups decreased by almost a half from day 3 to 4, which corresponded to the effect of one oral administration of **43M1** or **47M1**. The treatment groups displayed a relatively smaller population of trophozoites and schizonts compared to the untreated group on day 4. This suggests that **43M1** and **47M1** halted the development of trophozoites to schizonts. **43M1** and **47M1** are proposed to arrest the development of trophozoite-stage parasites that are actively catabolising haemoglobin which, therefore, prevents the formation of schizont-stage parasites. Consequently, the observed relative absence of trophozoite- and schizont-stage parasites on day 4 compared to the untreated control correlates well to the stage-specificity of **43M1** and **47M1**. Additionally, the reduction in phE from day 3 to 4 can be attributed to the parasiticidal activity of **43M1** and **47M1**, which inhibit haemozoin formation resulting in a toxic accumulation of FPIX[77]. The parasitaemia of the treatment groups on day 5, **Figure 4.6.H** and **M**, display a significantly smaller ring phase population compared to the untreated control on day 5. This can be attributed to the activity of **43M1** and **47M1** on trophozoite-stage parasites, which ultimately prevented the formation of schizonts on day 4, and therefore reduced the degree of parasite replication compared to the untreated control. On day 6, **Figure 4.6.I** and **N**, a pronounced absence of trophozoites and schizonts is displayed compared to the untreated control, which again can be as a result of the inhibitory effects of **43M1** and **47M1** on the development and growth of trophozoite-stage parasites. Day 7, **Figure 4.6.J** and **O**, displays the culmination of the gradual loss of ring-stage parasites due to the hindering effects of **43M1** and **47M1** on trophozoite-stage parasites, which consequently reduced parasite reinvasion and proliferation compared to the untreated control.

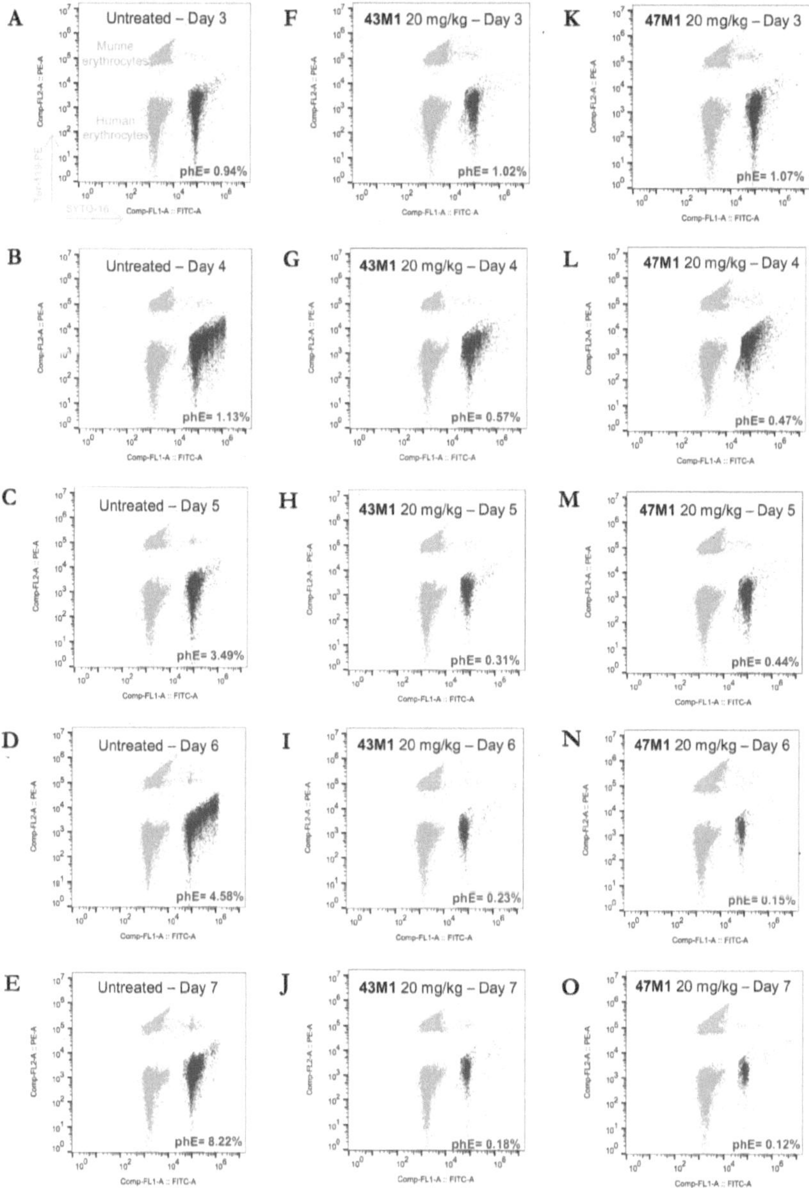

Figure 4.6. Representative flow cytometry dot plots of *P. falciparum*-infected chimeric peripheral blood of NSG mice displaying the morphological changes in the parasite populations from day 3–7 post infection after 4 daily consecutive oral administrations of **A-E** the oral dosing vehicle, **F-J** 20 mg/kg of **43M1**, and **K-O** 20 mg/kg of **47M1**.

The *in vivo* potency, or ED_{90}, of **43M1** and **47M1** in the *P. falciparum*-infected NSG murine model were 12 and 7.7 mg/kg, respectively. Their *in vivo* activity can be compared to that of several clinically relevant antimalarials which were tested in the same *in vivo* efficacy model of malaria. The activity of **43M1** is similar to lumefantrine (LUM), which exhibited an ED_{90} of 12 mg/kg; however, **43M1** was relatively less potent than artesunate, mefloquine (MEF), CQ, amodiaquine, piperaquine, pyrimethamine, and atovaquone (ATOV), which displayed ED_{90} values of 10, 7.7, 5, 4.2, 3.7, 0.9, and 0.05 mg/kg, respectively. The *in vivo* potency of **47M1** was comparable to that of MEF, and **47M1** displayed superior activity to artesunate and LUM and relatively lower activity compared to CQ, amodiaquine, piperaquine, pyrimethamine, and ATOV[171].

4.4. CONCLUSION

The PK/PD relationships which govern the *in vivo* antimalarial efficacy of **43M1** and **47M1** were determined in a *P. falciparum*-infected NSG murine model. **43M1** and **47M1** were efficacious against asexual intraerythrocytic *P. falciparum* *Pf*3D7$^{0087/N9}$ after 4 consecutive daily oral administrations of 20 mg/kg, which resulted in a 98% reduction in parasitaemia compared to the untreated group. Additionally, **43M1** and **47M1** displayed *in vivo* potencies of 12 and 7.7 mg/kg, respectively, which were within the range of other clinically relevant antimalarials. Given the promising *in vivo* antimalarial activity of **43M1** and **47M1**, these lead PBDQ compounds were further investigated to evaluate their potential to be used in combination therapy.

CHAPTER V

IN VITRO COMBINATIONS WITH CLINICALLY RELEVANT ANTIMALARIALS

5.1. INTRODUCTION

5.1.1. Chapter aim

This chapter investigates the *in vitro* interactions of the lead PDBQ candidates, **43M1** and **47M1**, in combination with clinically relevant antimalarials in CQS and CQR strains of *P. falciparum*. The purpose of this study was to identify synergistic combination partners with distinct drug targets, as this approach is expected to delay the evolution of resistance[16,172].

5.1.2. Combination therapy

As discussed in **Chapter I**, one of the major obstacles in malaria control is the recurring emergence and dissemination of drug-resistant strains. To overcome this hinderance, combination therapy has been clinically implemented, which utilises two or more antimalarials with unrelated drug targets as this is hypothesised to aid in delaying the appearance of resistance. Drug resistance occurs when parasites in a population exhibit spontaneous genetic mutations which decrease their drug susceptibility, and consequently allows their proliferation in the presence of treatment, especially when exposed to subtherapeutic drug concentrations[172]. The strategy behind combination therapy is to reduce the probability of resistant parasites emerging such that, if a parasite becomes resistant to one drug target, there is another drug which acts on a different target to which the parasite is still sensitive. This can ultimately delay the selection of successful mutant parasites and impede the propagation of resistant strains[173,174]. Furthermore, it is unlikely that parasites will simultaneously develop resistance against distinct drug targets as the mechanisms of resistance of two unrelated modes of action is theorised to be different[16]. In cases where synergy between drugs is exhibited, other benefits of combination therapy include improved therapeutic efficacy and subsequent potential dose and toxicity risk reduction[175,176]. Additionally, it is important to elucidate possible antagonistic drug interactions which could reduce therapeutic efficacy.

In general, synergy is a term used to describe the nature of the interaction of Drug A and Drug B where the activity of Drug A enhances the activity of Drug B and vice versa or, alternatively, when the combined effect of Drug A and Drug B is greater than the sum of the individual effects of Drug A and Drug B. The converse interaction is termed antagonism, where the activity of Drug A reduces the activity of Drug B and vice versa, or where the overall potency of the combination is less than the sum of their individual potencies. When a drug pair exhibits no enhancement or reduction in activity, and the combination potency remains unchanged relative to each drug alone, then the interaction reflects an additive or indifferent effect[177,178].

Synergy and antagonism occur as a result of molecular interactions between components of the biological targets of Drug A and Drug B, which in most cases is a protein or a biochemical pathway[177]. The interpretations of the interactions are dependent on the mechanisms of each drug and their resulting biochemical activities, which are often unknown and complex; therefore, there is no definitive method of predicting interactions based purely on different or similar mechanisms of action[177,179]. However, to aid in understanding the data presented in this chapter, a simplified explanation for the interactions is described below.

Synergy can occur when drugs exhibit similar mechanisms of action and bind at different sites on a common receptor or protein, in such a way that, for example, the binding of Drug A enhances the binding of Drug B. Additionally, synergy can be displayed when drugs have different mechanisms of action, but, for example, a product produced during the action of Drug A enhances the activity of Drug B and vice versa[177,179].

The opposite effect of synergy is described by antagonism, where drugs which exhibit similar mechanisms of action can display competitive inhibition by acting at the same site on a common receptor. Additionally, drugs with different mechanisms of action can also demonstrate antagonism if the activity of Drug A produces a product or interacts with a protein in such a way that it interferes with the activity of Drug B and vice versa[177,179].

Additivity can occur between drugs with independent and distinct modes of action; as well as with drugs which display similar modes of action but act in a non-competitive manner[177,179].

In vitro combination methods measure direct drug interactions; however, in an *in vivo* setting, drug interactions are influenced by differences in individual PK profiles and, therefore, there is a possibility that an *in vitro* interaction will not translate to a similar *in vivo* interaction. A specific example relates to two drugs with different elimination rates, for example, if Drug A has a fast elimination and Drug B is slowly eliminated, their mismatch in PK could result in monotherapy exposure of Drug B. Not only could this alter the interactions between Drug A and Drug B but additionally, it could provide selective pressure for the emergence of parasites resistant to Drug B[180]. Therefore, when combinations are considered, it is valuable to partner drugs with similar or complementary PK. However, the purpose of this study was to probe the potential of the PDBQ lead candidates to be used in combination therapy and, thus, for this preliminary investigation only PD differences were considered.

5.1.3. A short mechanistic review of selected antimalarial agents

5.1.3.1. Chloroquine

CQ, amodiaquine, and piperaquine belong to the quinoline class of antimalarials, as shown in **Figure 5.1**. In clinical use, amodiaquine and piperaquine are partnered with artesunate and DHA, respectively[15].

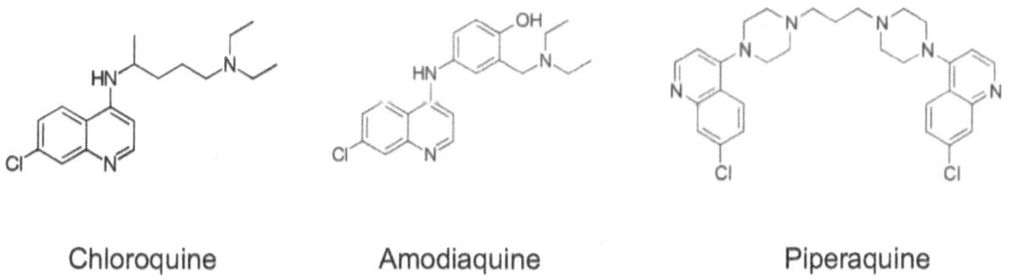

Chloroquine Amodiaquine Piperaquine

Figure 5.1. Chemical structures of CQ, amodiaquine, and piperaquine belonging to the quinoline class of compounds.

As discussed in **Chapter I**, quinolines exert their activity in the parasite DV through the inhibition of haemozoin formation resulting in FPIX-induced oxidative damage[181,182]. The PDBQ compounds act through a similar mechanism of action by inhibiting FPIX crystallisation to a degree comparable to that of CQ[77]. The SAR of CQ suggests that its antiplasmodial activity is dependent on the strength of FPIX binding, the degree of β-haematin inhibition, and the extent of accumulation within the DV[55]. Since the PDBQ compounds conserve the CQ pharmacophore, the PDBQ metabolites are hypothesised to exhibit a SAR similar to that of CQ. Although the stage specificity of the PDBQ metabolites has not yet been investigated, they are proposed to act during the trophozoite stage when haemoglobin uptake and digestion is at its peak[183,184]. CQ resistance is mediated by point mutations in the drug transporter PfCRT which, in resistant strains, is able to efflux CQ out of the DV thus extruding it from its site of action[59,182]. The reduced accumulation of CQ within the DV of CQR strains allows the parasite to control the FPIX detoxification process[64]. Mutations in another DV transporter protein, PfMDR1, has also been implicated in modulating CQ resistance, but specifically in strains which possess the CQR PfCRT genetic background[185]. The PDBQ metabolites do not share cross-resistance with CQ[77].

5.1.3.2. Dihydroartemisinin

DHA is the primary active metabolite of ART and its synthetic derivatives, artesunate and artemether. Artemisinins are classified as sesquiterpene lactones and contain an endoperoxide group, as shown in **Figure 5.2**.

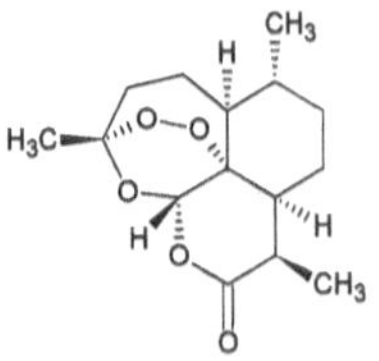

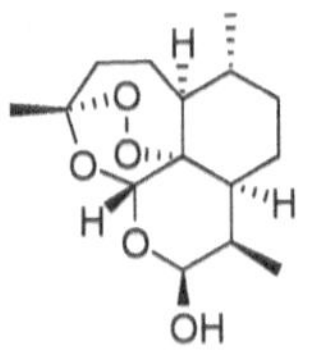

Artemisinin

Dihydroartemisinin

Figure 5.2. Chemical structures of the endoperoxides ART and its active metabolite DHA.

Artemisinins are fast-acting against the asexual intraerythrocytic stages of the *P. falciparum* lifecycle, however, they are rapidly eliminated. Therefore, to mitigate the risk of recrudescence, artemisinins are partnered with a relatively slow-acting antimalarial which exhibits a longer elimination phase[15]. ART and DHA exert their activity through their endoperoxide pharmacophore. In order to initiate drug activation, the endoperoxide bridge is theorised to be cleaved either by FPIX or by free Fe(II). When in contact with FPIX or Fe(II), the endoperoxide ring cleaves producing free radicals which induce oxidative stress in the parasite and cause protein damage[186,187,188]. Additionally, activated DHA and ART have been shown to bind to numerous target sites, suggesting multiple modes of action, including the inhibition of *P. falciparum* phosphatidylinositol-3-kinase[189,190]. Artemisinins exhibit a broad stage specificity of action. They act on ring-stage parasites, including young rings as well as trophozoite-phase parasites[184,191]. Although the mechanism of ART resistance is still unclear, it has been associated with mutations in *pfkelch13*[192].

5.1.3.3. Mefloquine

MEF is an aryl amino alcohol and is illustrated in **Figure 5.3**.

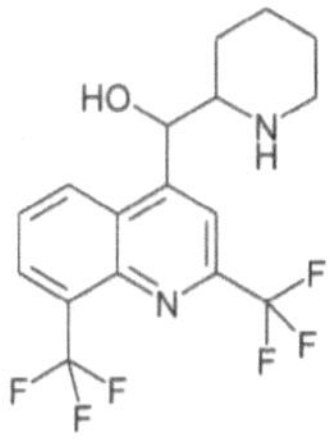

Figure 5.3. Chemical structure of MEF.

MEF is used clinically in combination with artesunate for treatment against CQS and CQR strains of *P. falciparum*[15]. MEF acts during the asexual intraerythrocytic stages of the *P. falciparum* lifecycle, specifically against mid- to late-trophozoite parasites. MEF is a weak inhibitor of haemozoin formation which suggests that it exerts its antimalarial activity through alternative modes of action[181,193]. MEF has been shown to bind to the cytoplasmic 80S ribosome of *P. falciparum*, which results in the inhibition of parasite protein synthesis[194]. MEF resistance is associated with an increase in the copy number of the drug transporter P-glycoprotein homologue-1, or Pgh-1, which is encoded by *pfmdr1*. In MEF-resistant strains, Pgh-1 effluxes MEF from the parasite cytosol into the DV, which further supports the proposal that haemozoin inhibition is not the primary mechanism of action, as MEF antimalarial activity does not appear to increase even in the presence of higher concentrations of MEF in the DV of resistant strains[65,185,195,196].

5.1.3.4. Lumefantrine

LUM is a fluorene derivative of the aryl amino alcohols, illustrated in **Figure 5.4**, and belongs to the same class of compounds as MEF.

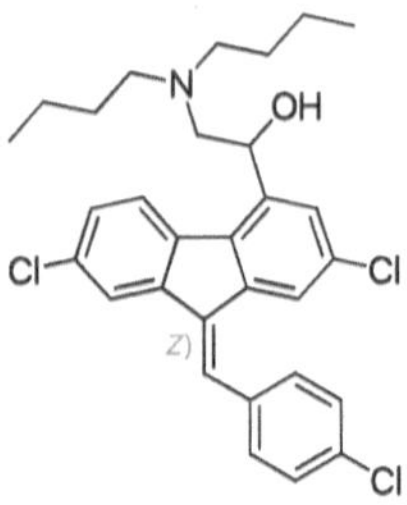

Figure 5.4. Chemical structure of LUM.

LUM is used clinically in combination with artemether[15]. It is active against the asexual intraerythrocytic stages of the *P. falciparum* lifecycle[193]. Although the exact mechanism of action of LUM has not yet been fully characterised, experimental evidence suggests that it weakly arrests the FPIX detoxification pathway, amongst other unknown primary modes of action which are postulated to occur within the parasite cytosol[181,197]. A marker for LUM resistance is the amplification of the *pfmdr1* copy number[198,199].

5.1.3.5. Methylene blue

Methylene blue (MB) is a thiazine dye and is illustrated in **Figure 5.5**.

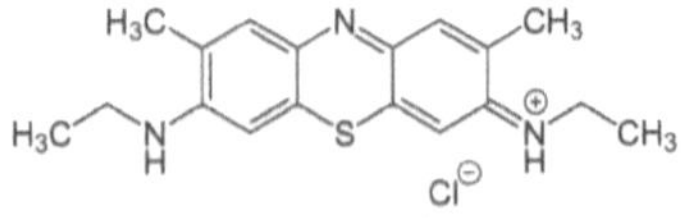

Figure 5.5. Chemical structure of MB.

MB has been shown to induce oxidative stress by specifically inhibiting *P. falciparum* glutathione reductase (GR), which is involved in the redox balance control system of the parasite[200,201]. Although MB is active against all blood stages of the *P. falciparum* lifecycle, the ring and early-trophozoite phases were shown to be the most susceptible to MB activity, and late trophozoites and schizonts displayed reduced sensitivity towards MB[202,203]. Resistance to MB has not yet become apparent, and it has been observed that MB resistance is difficult to induce in an *in vivo* animal model[204]. Although MB is currently not used clinically, there has been growing interest to reintroduce it for antimalarial therapy[203,205].

5.1.3.6. Atovaquone

ATOV is a hydroxynaphthoquinone derivative and is displayed in **Figure 5.6.**

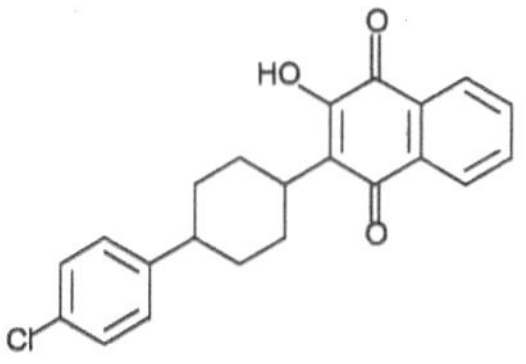

Figure 5.6. Chemical structure of ATOV.

ATOV interrupts the parasite mitochondrial electron transport system by inhibiting the cytochrome *bc_1* complex which is involved in the transduction of energy[206,207]. The binding of ATOV to cytochrome *bc_1* impairs pyrimidine synthesis[208]. ATOV displays a slow onset of action by acting on late trophozoites undergoing DNA replication[191,193]. ATOV resistance is mediated through mutations on the ATOV binding site of *cytochrome b*[209].

5.1.4. Fixed-dose ratio isobolograms

There is no standardised method to assess *in vitro* interactions between drugs. Various techniques and models have been developed to study *in vitro* drug combinations such as the checkerboard method, the Chou-Talalay method, and the isobologram method, the last of which has been adopted in this study[210,211,212,213,214].

The isobologram method, using a fixed-dose ratio procedure, determines the combined activity of Drug A and Drug B at various concentration ratios of each drug. The interactions between Drug A and Drug B might differ depending on the concentration of each drug in the combination, therefore, a range of concentration ratios is often used specifically, 5:0,

4:1, 3:2, 2:3, 1:4, and 0:5 of Drug A to Drug B. In order to generate a dose-response curve for each drug at each combination ratio, a range of concentrations need to be tested which encompass maximal and minimal growth inhibition. This concentration range is usually achieved by serially diluting a starting concentration to cover at least eight concentration values. This method is referred to as a fixed-ratio procedure because for each combination ratio, the serial dilutions are prepared to allow a constant ratio of Drug A and Drug B over the dosing range. The ratios of each drug in a combination represent fractions of each compound's respective IC_{50}[215].

Each combination generates two dose-response curves, as they use the same inhibition data but cover different concentration ranges, which are determined by the starting concentration of each drug in the combination. The combination ratios of 5:0 and 0:5 of Drug A to Drug B establish the IC_{50} of each drug alone, and these values are used as a baseline for individual activity. When comparing the IC_{50} of Drug A or Drug B in combination to its IC_{50} alone, if the IC_{50} decreases in combination compared to its individual IC_{50} then, this is reflective of a synergistic interaction. If the IC_{50} increases in combination compared to its individual IC_{50} then, this is reflective of an antagonistic interaction. Lastly, if the IC_{50} is similar when used alone and when used in combination, it indicates an indifferent or additive interaction[215,216].

To numerically define the interaction between Drug A and Drug B, the activity of each drug alone is compared to the activity of each drug in combination using the fractional IC_{50} (FIC_{50}) as shown in **Equation 5.1** and **Equation 5.2** below.

$$FIC_{50} \text{ of Drug A} = \frac{IC_{50} \text{ of Drug A in combination}}{IC_{50} \text{ of Drug A alone}}$$ **Equation 5.1**

$$FIC_{50} \text{ of Drug B} = \frac{IC_{50} \text{ of Drug B in combination}}{IC_{50} \text{ of Drug B alone}}$$ **Equation 5.2**

The sum of the fractional IC_{50} values (ΣFIC_{50}) at each combination ratio is defined as the sum of the FIC_{50} of Drug A and the FIC_{50} of Drug B and indicates the nature of the interaction at the specific fixed-ratio. The overall extent of the interaction of the drug combination is quantitatively defined as the overall mean ΣFIC_{50}, which is determined by averaging the ΣFIC_{50} values of each fixed-ratio combination[215,216,217]. There is no harmonised definition for the interactions represented by the ΣFIC_{50} values. For the purposes of this study, the following classification index was adopted based on values presented in literature. ΣFIC_{50} values less than 0.8 indicate synergism, ΣFIC_{50} values between 0.8–1.4 indicate additivity, and ΣFIC_{50} values above 1.4 indicate antagonism[218,219].

An isobologram is used to graphically represent the nature of the interactions between Drug A and Drug B. An explanatory isobologram is presented in **Figure 5.7**. The x- and y-axes represent the FIC_{50} values of Drug A and Drug B, respectively at each fixed-ratio combination. The FIC_{50} of each drug alone is 1, and these values are plotted on each respective axis, the line which joins these two points depicts the isobole or the line of additivity and represents the effect of the individual drug[215,216].

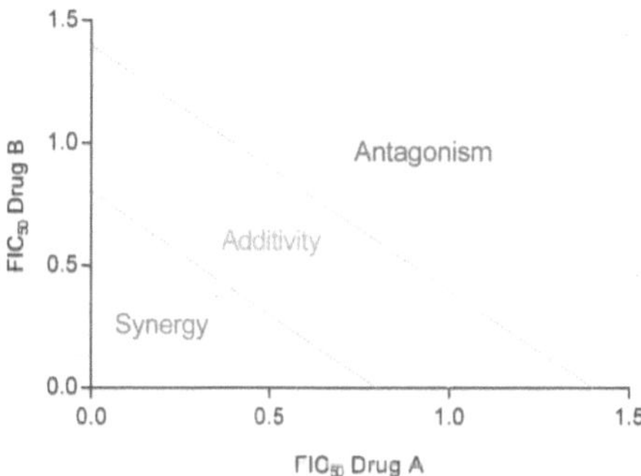

Figure 5.7. Isobologram illustrating the ranges of synergistic, additive, and antagonistic interactions of Drugs A and B in combination, as determined by their respective FIC_{50} values.

5.1.5. *In vitro* antimalarial isobologram study design

As discussed in **Chapter III** and **Chapter IV**, **43M1** and **47M1** displayed favourable *in vivo* antimalarial efficacy and were, therefore, chosen for further investigation to evaluate their potential to be used in combination therapy with clinical drugs of proven antimalarial efficacy. Additionally, the CQ-resistance reversing potential of **43M1** and **47M1**, as well as their respective parent compound, were evaluated.

The CQ-resistance reversing ability of selected PDBQ compounds were evaluated in the CQR strain *Pf*Dd2. The lead PDBQ compounds were tested in combination with the established antimalarials DHA, MEF, LUM, MB, and ATOV, all of which display dissimilar mechanisms of action to haemozoin inhibition. Each combination was tested against the CQS strain *Pf*NF54 and the CQR strain *Pf*Dd2. *Pf*NF54 has a wildtype PfCRT whereas *Pf*Dd2 possesses point mutations in PfCRT, amongst other associated mutations in PfMDR1[220,221]. Additionally, there is always a possibility of unknown drug transporter mutations that could have arisen during continuous culturing; nonetheless, the single compound growth inhibition assay was able to demonstrate the drug susceptibility in each strain.

Other quinoline antimalarials, which share a common mode of action to the PDBQ compounds, were excluded from this study as they are proposed to be unsuitable combination partners. Furthermore, although the antifolates act on a distinct drug target to FPIX, they were not included in this study as the *in vitro* malaria culture medium contains folate which can be utilised by the parasite.

5.2. METHODS

The following section summarises the methods used for the *in vitro* antimalarial combination studies. A complete description of the materials used in this chapter is presented in **Appendix C**. All techniques and assays were performed under sterile conditions, unless otherwise stated.

5.2.1. *In vitro* continuous culture of *Plasmodium falciparum*

Strains of *P. falciparum* were continuously cultured *in vitro* using a modified method described by Trager and Jensen[222]. In summary, parasites were maintained at a 2% haematocrit in washed O+ human erythrocytes and complete medium. The parasitaemia and predominant phase of the culture were determined daily by viewing samples of the culture under light microscopy. In order to accurately measure the parasitaemia, a total of at least 500 erythrocytes were counted. Briefly, culture blood smears were fixed with MeOH and stained with 10% (v/v) Giesma in PBS before being viewed under an oil immersion lens. Trophozoite cultures were diluted with washed O+ human erythrocytes to maintain a 2% haematocrit and 5% parasitaemia. Ring-phase cultures were synchronised with 5 volumes of 5% (w/v) D-sorbitol in H_2O for 10 min at 37°C. The culture volume was maintained at 40 ml in a 200 ml culture flask. Cultures were incubated at 37°C under a gas environment of 3% O_2, 4% CO_2, and 93% N_2[222,223].

5.2.2. *In vitro* antiplasmodial assays

The parasite lactate dehydrogenase (pLDH) assay was used to determine the *in vitro* antiplasmodial activity of single compounds and combinations using a modified method described by Makler and Hinrichs[224]. The pLDH assay is a colourimetric, enzymatic assay which indirectly measures malaria parasite growth and survival. During glycolysis pLDH, which is present in both the malaria parasite and erythrocyte, converts lactate to pyruvate using nicotinamide adenine dinucleotide (NAD) as a coenzyme. NAD activity in the parasite is indistinguishable from that in the erythrocyte but, the NAD analogue, 3-acetyl pyridine dinucleotide (APAD), is specific to the parasite. APAD is reduced to APADH during glycolysis in living parasites. The pLDH assay uses yellow coloured nitroblue tetrazolium (NBT), and during the conversion of lactate to pyruvate, APADH reduces yellow NBT to a purple formazan salt. During plate development, parasites are supplemented with APAD, lactate, and NBT. Living parasites are able to reduce APAD at a higher rate compared to the erythrocyte. Therefore, the rate of NBT conversion and consequently, the degree of colour change from yellow to purple corresponds to the number of living parasites. The colour change intensities are measured by absorption spectroscopy at 620 nm, and this correlates to the changes in parasite growth and survival over the tested concentration range[224]. The pLDH plate development procedure was performed under non-sterile conditions

5.2.2.1. Single compound antiplasmodial assay

The antiplasmodial activity of each compound tested in the combination experiments was determined in *Pf*NF54 and *Pf*Dd2 over two independent assays, each performed in triplicate (n = 6). Each assay was prepared with CQ as a positive control. On the day of the experiment, drug stock solutions were prepared to 2 mg/ml in DMSO. The test drug stock solution was then diluted with complete medium to starting concentrations of 200 and 2000 ng/ml. One hundred microlitres of each starting concentration solution was plated in triplicate in a flat-bottom 96-well microtiter plate. The starting concentrations were then serially diluted twofold with complete medium to cover an overall concentration range from 0.2–1000 ng/ml. Each plate was prepared with a blank column which contained 100 µl of unparasitised erythrocytes at a 2% haematocrit in complete medium, and a drug-free positive control column which contained 100 µl of trophozoite-phase parasitised erythrocytes at a 2% haematocrit and 2% parasitaemia. Additionally, 100 µl of trophozoite-phase parasites at a 2% haematocrit and 2% parasitaemia were added to each drug testing well. The plate was incubated at 37°C under a gas environment of 3% O_2, 4% CO_2, and 93% N_2 for one 48 h parasite lifecycle[222,224].

Following incubation, the erythrocytes underwent freeze-thaw lysis, and then the plate was developed using the following pLDH method. 15 µl of resuspended erythrocytes were added to 100 µl of Malstat, containing APAD and calcium L-lactate hydrate, and 15 µl of NBT[224]. The plate was place in the dark to develop, and then the absorbance of each well was measured at 620 nm using the Modulus Microplate Multimode Reader (Turner Biosystems, Inc., California, US). The IC_{50} value was determined by fitting the

log_{10}(concentration) and blank corrected absorbance values to a non-linear dose-response curve using GraphPad Prism software version 4 (GraphPad Software Inc., California, US).

5.2.2.2. Fixed-ratio isobologram assay

The combination experiments were performed using a modified fixed-ratio isobologram method described by Fivelman, Adagu, and Warhurst[215]. Each combination was tested with two independent biological replicates each prepared in triplicate (n = 6). A control fixed-dose ratio isobologram assay was first performed to validate the experimental procedure (data not shown). The interaction of either **43M1** or **47M1**, hereafter referred to as Drug A, with a clinically relevant antimalarial, hereafter referred to as Drug B, was determined in both *Pf*NF54 and *Pf*Dd2. The determined individual IC_{50} values of Drug A and Drug B served as a positive control for each assay.

On the day of the experiment, drug stock solutions were prepared in DMSO at 2 mg/ml. Dilutions of the stock solutions of Drug A and Drug B were prepared with complete medium to starting concentrations of 6 times each test compound's predetermined individual IC_{50} value, namely solution A for Drug A and solution B for Drug B. This 6 times starting concentration solution was made to allow the experimental IC_{50} to fall around the fourth twofold serial dilution or midway down the plate. The drug combination solutions were prepared with Solution A and Solution B, according to the combination ratios presented in **Table 5.1**. For example, Solution 2 was prepared by mixing 4 parts of Solution A with 1 part of Solution B, resulting in a 4 in 5 dilution of the starting concentration of Solution A and a 1 in 5 dilution of the starting concentration of Solution B.

Table 5.1. Explanatory table describing the plating concentrations of the combination of Drug A and Drug B using the fixed-ratio isobologram method. The starting concentrations of Solution A and Solution B are prepared to 6 times the respective IC_{50} of Drug A and Drug B. The drugs are assigned arbitrary IC_{50} values of 10 and 15 mg/ml for Drug A and Drug B, respectively.

Combination solution	Ratio of Drug A to Drug B	Final plating concentration (ng/ml)	
		Drug A	Drug B
Solution 1	5:0	60	0
Solution 2	4:1	48	18
Solution 3	3:2	36	36
Solution 4	2:3	24	54
Solution 5	1:4	12	72
Solution 6	0:5	0	90

One hundred microlitres of each drug combination solution for each ratio was plated in triplicate over two flat-bottom 96-well microtiter plates and serially diluted twofold, down the plate, with complete medium to maintain fixed-ratios to cover a range of 8 concentrations, as displayed by **Figure 5.8**.

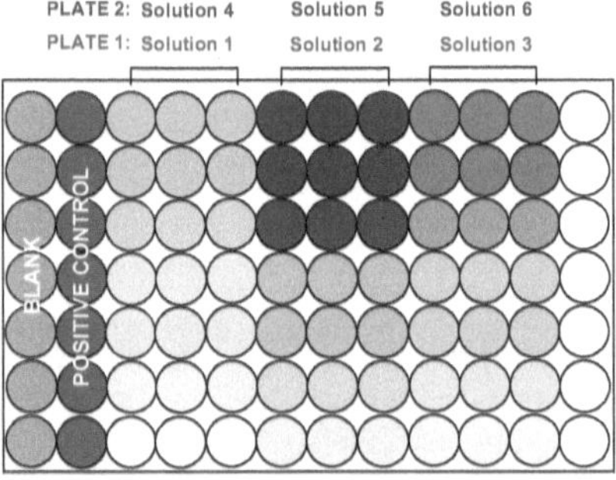

Figure 5.8. Representative plating procedure for the fixed-ratio isobolograms for the combination of Drug A and Drug B. Solutions 1 to 6 represent different concentration ratios of Drug A to Drug B which are serially diluted twofold, down the plate, and maintained at constant ratios.

Each plate was prepared with a blank column which contained 100 µl of unparasitised erythrocytes at a 2% haematocrit in complete medium, and a positive control column which contained 100 µl of trophozoite-phase parasitised erythrocytes at a 2% haematocrit and 2% parasitaemia. Additionally, each combination testing well received 100 µl of the parasitised erythrocyte suspension of a 2% haematocrit and 2% parasitaemia. The plate was incubated at 37°C under a gas environment of 3% O_2, 4% CO_2, and 93% N_2 for 48 h[215,222]. After incubation and freeze-thaw lysis, the plates were developed using the pLDH assay, as previously described in **Section 5.2.2.1**.

The IC_{50}s of Drug A and Drug B alone and the two IC_{50} values for each drug in each combination ratio were determined by fitting the respective log_{10}(concentration) and blank-corrected absorbance values to a non-linear dose-response curve using GraphPad Prism version 4 software. Dose-response curves for each drug in each combination were generated. The FIC_{50} for each drug at each combination ratio was calculated by dividing the apparent IC_{50} of the drug in combination with the IC_{50} of the drug alone, as shown in **Equation 5.1** and **Equation 5.2**. The ΣFIC_{50} value for each combination ratio was determined by adding the respective FIC_{50} values of Drug A and Drug B. The overall interaction of the combination was determined by averaging the ΣFIC_{50} values of each combination ratio. All FIC_{50} calculations were performed in Microsoft Excel version 16.31 (Microsoft Corporation, Washington, US). All values are reported as the mean ± SEM.

As previously discussed in **Section 5.1.4**, a ΣFIC_{50} value less than 0.8 indicates synergism, a ΣFIC_{50} value between 0.8–1.4 reflects an additive or indifferent interaction, and a ΣFIC_{50} value greater than 1.4 indicates antagonism[218,219]. These threshold values were set to account for experimental error due to biological variability. The isobologram was plotted using the mean FIC_{50} of Drug A against the mean FIC_{50} of Drug B at each combination ratio in GraphPad Prism software version 4. The isobolograms did not include the error bars associated with the means, but, in **Section 5.3**, the experimental variability (SEM) of these values is presented in the numerical interaction data tables which summarises the FIC_{50} and ΣFIC_{50} data.

5.3. RESULTS AND DISCUSSION

5.3.1. Single compound antiplasmodial activity

Table 5.2 displays the single compound antiplasmodial activity of selected antimalarials in CQS *Pf*NF54 and CQR *Pf*Dd2. **43M1, 47M1,** and all clinical drugs displayed favourable activity against *Pf*NF54 and *Pf*Dd2. Since *Pf*Dd2 is a CQR strain, CQ showed decreased activity in *Pf*Dd2 compared to its activity in *Pf*NF54.

Table 5.2. *In vitro* drug susceptibilities of clinically relevant antimalarials, **36**, and selected PDBQ compounds in CQS *Pf*NF54 and CQR *Pf*Dd2[a]

Drug	IC_{50} (nM)[b,c]	
	***Pf*NF54**	***Pf*Dd2**
DHA	0.8 ± 0.1	3 ± 1
MEF	9 ± 2	5 ± 2
LUM	2 ± 1	1.9 ± 0.7
MB	5.7 ± 0.5	10 ± 2
ATOV	1.3 ± 0.5	12 ± 2
CQ	9 ± 1	177 ± 6
36	12 ± 2	32 ± 2
43	25 ± 2	103 ± 5
43M1	6 ± 1	48 ± 2
47	45 ± 2	139 ± 3
47M1	5 ± 1	37 ± 2

[a]IC_{50} values derived from a 48 h pLDH assay. [b]Values presented as the mean ± SEM. [c]$4 \leq n \leq 6$.

5.3.2. Combinations with chloroquine

The CQ-resistance reversing potential of **43M1** and **47M1**, and their respective parents, were assessed in the CQR strain *Pf*Dd2, as presented in **Figure 5.9, Figure 5.10, Table 5.3**, and **Table 5.4**. Since the DBQ compound **36** has been shown to reverse CQ resistance by directly inhibiting CQ transport by the CQR PfCRT, the interactions of the PDBQ compounds with CQ were compared to that of **36** with CQ[74]. The isobolograms illustrate synergistic interactions between CQ and the parent PDBQ compound, **43** or **47**, at all combination ratios in the CQR strain. The interactions of **43** or **47** with CQ are comparable to those of CQ with **36**, where all combinations displayed mean FIC_{50} values below the line of additivity. The PDBQ metabolites, **43M1** and **47M1**, however, displayed an overall additive relationship with CQ in the CQR strain as displayed by the mean FIC_{50} values which are generally within the additivity region of the isobologram.

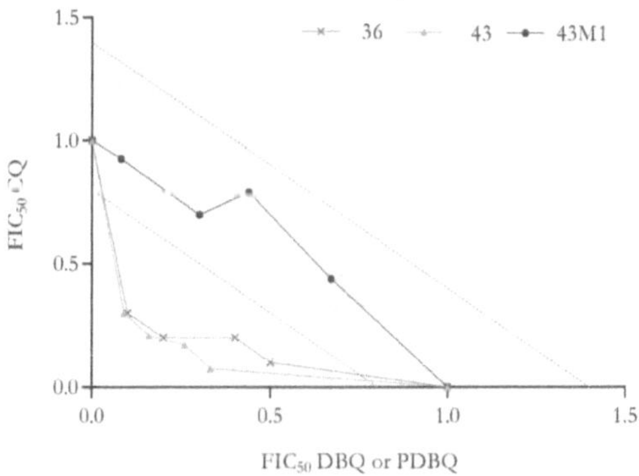

Figure 5.9. Isobologram illustrating the *in vitro* interactions of **36**, **43**, or **43M1** with CQ in CQR *Pf*Dd2 using a fixed-ratio procedure (FIC_{50} values presented as the mean, n = 6).

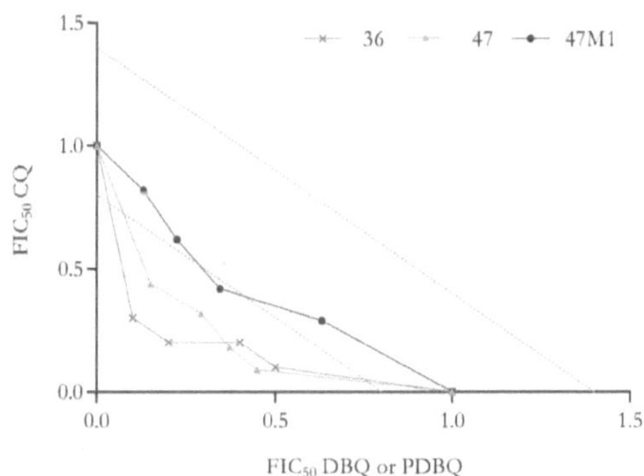

Figure 5.10. Isobologram illustrating the *in vitro* interactions of **36**, **47**, or **47M1** with CQ in CQR *Pf*Dd2 using a fixed-ratio procedure (FIC_{50} values presented as the mean, n = 6).

As displayed in **Table 5.3** and **Table 5.4**, the overall mean ΣFIC_{50} values of **43** or **47** with CQ in *Pf*Dd2 were 0.40 ± 0.01 and 0.57 ± 0.02, respectively and the overall mean ΣFIC_{50}

values of **43M1** or **47M1** with CQ in *Pf*Dd2 were 1.09 ± 0.05 and 0.87 ± 0.04, respectively. The mean ΣFIC_{50} values further reflect the overall synergy between the PDBQ parents and CQ and the overall additivity between the M1 PDBQ metabolites and CQ.

Table 5.3. *In vitro* antimalarial interactions of **43** or **43M1** with CQ against CQR *Pf*Dd2 using a fixed-ratio isobologram method[a]

Combination ratio of PDBQ:CQ	Mean ± SEM FIC_{50}[b]			
	*Pf*Dd2		*Pf*Dd2	
	43	CQ	43M1	CQ
4:1	0.33 ± 0.05	0.076 ± 0.003	0.67 ± 0.04	0.44 ± 0.02
3:2	0.26 ± 0.06	0.17 ± 0.03	0.44 ± 0.03	0.79 ± 0.02
2:3	0.16 ± 0.05	0.21 ± 0.05	0.30 ± 0.09	0.7 ± 0.2
1:4	0.09 ± 0.02	0.30 ± 0.03	0.082 ± 0.006	0.926 ± 0.001
Overall mean ΣFIC_{50} ± SEM	0.40 ± 0.01		1.09 ± 0.05	
Overall interaction	Synergistic		Additive	

[a]IC_{50} values derived using a 48 h pLDH assay. [b]$n = 6$.

Table 5.4. *In vitro* antimalarial interactions of **47** or **47M1** with CQ against CQR *Pf*Dd2 using a fixed-ratio isobologram method[a]

Combination ratio of PDBQ:CQ	Mean ± SEM FIC_{50}[b]			
	*Pf*Dd2		*Pf*Dd2	
	47	CQ	47M1	CQ
4:1	0.45 ± 0.08	0.09 ± 0.03	0.63 ± 0.06	0.29 ± 0.07
3:2	0.37 ± 0.09	0.18 ± 0.01	0.343 ± 0.004	0.42 ± 0.07
2:3	0.29 ± 0.04	0.32 ± 0.01	0.223 ± 0.005	0.62 ± 0.07
1:4	0.15 ± 0.06	0.44 ± 0.09	0.13 ± 0.02	0.83 ± 0.07
Overall mean ΣFIC_{50} ± SEM	0.57 ± 0.02		0.87 ± 0.04	
Overall interaction	Synergistic		Additive	

[a]IC_{50} values derived using a 48 h pLDH assay. [b]$n = 6$.

The synergistic interactions between **43** or **47** and CQ are hypothesised to be comparable to the synergistic interactions between **36** and CQ. The dibenzylmethylamine side chain of the DBQ **36** has been shown to inhibit the transport of CQ by the CQR PfCRT. This relationship has been directly demonstrated using isobologram analyses and the *X. laevis* oocyte PfCRT expression system[74]. The modified dibenzylmethylamine side chain of the PDBQ parent compound is theorised to interact with the CQR PfCRT in a similar manner to that of **36**, which ultimately promotes the accumulation of CQ at its site of action within the DV. These observed synergistic interactions, therefore, suggest that **43** and **47** are able to chemosensitise CQR strains.

43M1 and **47M1**, however, displayed an overall additive interaction with CQ in the resistant strain, which suggests that they were unable to reverse CQ resistance in *Pf*Dd2. This is hypothesised to be as a result of the cleaved dibenzylmethylamine side chain of the M1 metabolite which now no longer has the structural characteristics required for it to inhibit CQ egress by CQR PfCRT. The lack of hindering interaction with PfCRT allows CQ efflux from the DV, thereby reducing the accumulation of CQ at its site of action.

Together these results suggest that the CQ chemosensitising activity of the PDBQ parent is not conserved in the M1 metabolite. Furthermore, the combination of **43M1** or **47M1** with CQ should not be used as a strategy to reverse CQ resistance as these metabolites were unable to potentiate the antiplasmodial activity of CQ in the CQR strain.

5.3.3. Combinations with dihydroartemisinin

Figure 5.11, **Figure 5.12**, **Table 5.5**, and **Table 5.6** present the *in vitro* antimalarial interactions of **43M1** or **47M1** in combination with DHA in *Pf*NF54 and *Pf*Dd2. The isobolograms illustrate synergistic interactions between **43M1** or **47M1** and DHA at all combination ratios in both the CQS and CQR strains. This is demonstrated by the mean FIC_{50} values which all lie below the lower limit of additivity.

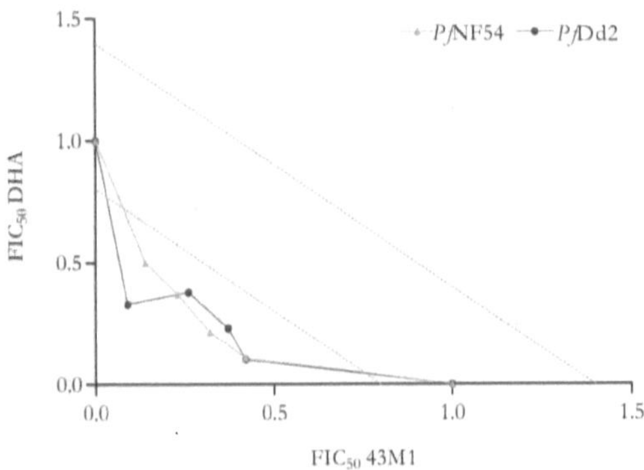

Figure 5.11. Isobologram illustrating the *in vitro* interactions of **43M1** with DHA in CQS *Pf*NF54 and CQR *Pf*Dd2 using a fixed-ratio procedure (FIC_{50} values presented as the mean, $n = 6$).

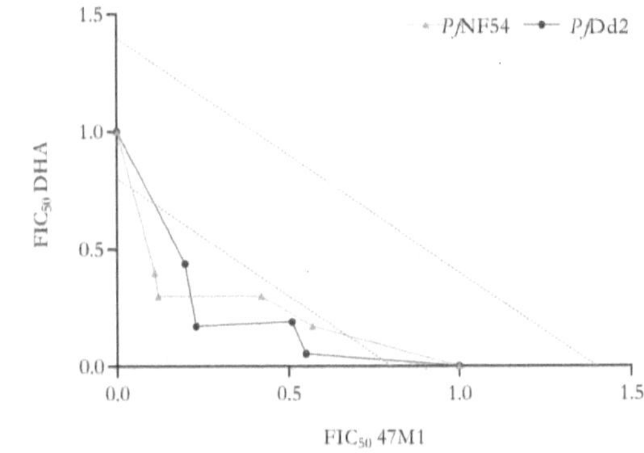

Figure 5.12. Isobologram illustrating the *in vitro* interactions of **47M1** with DHA in CQS *Pf*NF54 and CQR *Pf*Dd2 using a fixed-ratio procedure (FIC_{50} values presented as the mean, $n = 6$).

As summarised in **Table 5.5** and **Table 5.6** the synergistic interactions between **43M1** or **47M1** and DHA are further supported by the overall mean ΣFIC_{50} values, which were below the limit of additivity of 0.8. **43M1** and DHA displayed synergistic overall mean ΣFIC_{50} values of 0.58 ± 0.03 and 0.55 ± 0.05 in *Pf*NF54 and *Pf*Dd2, respectively. Additionally, **47M1** and DHA displayed comparable synergistic interactions with overall mean ΣFIC_{50}

values of 0.60 ± 0.08 in *Pf*NF54 and 0.54 ± 0.06 in *Pf*Dd2. **43M1** and **47M1** displayed similar degrees of synergism with DHA in both the CQS and CQR strains. The dose-ratios of 3:2 and 4:1 of **43M1** to DHA displayed the greatest relative potentiation in antimalarial activity in *Pf*NF54 compared to the other dosing ratios. In *Pf*Dd2, the dosing ratio of 1:4 of **43M1** to DHA displayed the highest relative synergistic effect compared to the other dosing ratios. The dosing ratio of 2:3 of **47M1** to DHA achieved the highest synergistic activity in both *Pf*NF54 and *Pf*Dd2 compared to the other dosing ratios.

Table 5.5. *In vitro* antimalarial interactions of **43M1** with DHA against CQS *Pf*NF54 and CQR *Pf*Dd2 using a fixed-ratio isobologram method[a]

Combination ratio of 43M1:DHA	Mean ± SEM FIC_{50}[b]			
	***Pf*NF54**		***Pf*Dd2**	
	43M1	**DHA**	**43M1**	**DHA**
4:1	0.419 ± 0.006	0.11 ± 0.02	0.42 ± 0.03	0.102 ± 0.008
3:2	0.32 ± 0.06	0.216 ± 0.006	0.37 ± 0.04	0.23 ± 0.01
2:3	0.23 ± 0.01	0.37 ± 0.05	0.26 ± 0.01	0.38 ± 0.04
1:4	0.14 ± 0.02	0.5 ± 0.2	0.09 ± 0.04	0.33 ± 0.09
Overall mean ΣFIC_{50} ± SEM	0.58 ± 0.03		0.55 ± 0.05	
Overall interaction	Synergistic		Synergistic	

[a]IC_{50} values derived using a 48 h pLDH assay. [b]$n = 6$.

Table 5.6. *In vitro* antimalarial interactions of **47M1** with DHA against CQS *Pf*NF54 and CQR *Pf*Dd2 using a fixed-ratio isobologram method[a]

Combination ratio of 47M1:DHA	Mean ± SEM FIC$_{50}$[b]			
	*Pf*NF54		*Pf*Dd2	
	47M1	**DHA**	**47M1**	**DHA**
4:1	0.57 ± 0.04	0.17 ± 0.08	0.55 ± 0.05	0.054 ± 0.002
3:2	0.42 ± 0.04	0.3 ± 0.1	0.51 ± 0.01	0.19 ± 0.01
2:3	0.12 ± 0.02	0.3 ± 0.2	0.23 ± 0.03	0.17 ± 0.02
1:4	0.11 ± 0.06	0.41 ± 0.03	0.199 ± 0.008	0.44 ± 0.04
Overall mean ΣFIC$_{50}$ ± SEM	0.60 ± 0.08		0.54 ± 0.06	
Overall interaction	Synergistic		Synergistic	

[a]IC$_{50}$ values derived using a 48 h pLDH assay. [b]n = 6.

The CQ resistance mechanisms did not appear to influence the interactions of **43M1** or **47M1** with DHA, as comparable synergy was displayed in both the CQS and CQR strains of *P. falciparum*. The synergistic observations are theorised to be based on the mechanism by which DHA is activated. The PDBQ metabolites act through the inhibition of haemozoin formation leading to an accumulation of FPIX. When used in combination, the presence of increased levels of FPIX presumably coincided with a more efficient activation of DHA through the FPIX-mediated catalysed scission of the endoperoxide bridge, which consequently resulted in the enhanced potency of DHA[225,226]. This theory is supported by the low mean FIC$_{50}$ values of DHA, especially when combined with higher concentrations of the haemozoin inhibitor when high levels of FPIX are expected to be present. Additionally, the synergism between **43M1** or **47M1** and DHA suggests that there was no competitive binding between the haemozoin inhibitor and DHA for the FPIX produced during haemoglobin catabolism[227].

43M1 or **47M1** with DHA revealed promising *in vitro* interactions, in addition to displaying distinct modes of action which can encourage the evasion of drug resistance, they were able to potentiate *in vitro* antimalarial activity which could potentially translate to enhanced efficacy.

5.3.4. Combinations with mefloquine

Figure 5.13, **Figure 5.14**, **Table 5.7**, and **Table 5.8** present the *in vitro* antimalarial interactions of **43M1** or **47M1** in combination with MEF against CQS *Pf*NF54 and CQR *Pf*Dd2. The isobolograms illustrate synergistic interactions in the CQS strain as shown by the mean FIC_{50} values, which all lie below the lower limit of additivity. However, this synergistic interaction was not reproduced in the CQR strain as **43M1** and **47M1** predominately acted antagonistically with MEF. The mean FIC_{50} values of this combination in *Pf*Dd2 were primarily above the upper limit of additivity except at one fixed-dose ratio where the mean FIC_{50} values were within the range of an indifferent interaction.

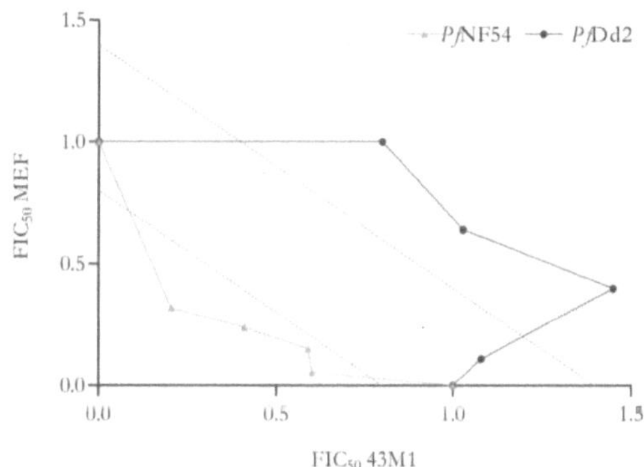

Figure 5.13. Isobologram illustrating the *in vitro* interactions of **43M1** with MEF in CQS *Pf*NF54 and CQR *Pf*Dd2 using a fixed-ratio procedure (FIC_{50} values presented as the mean, $n = 6$).

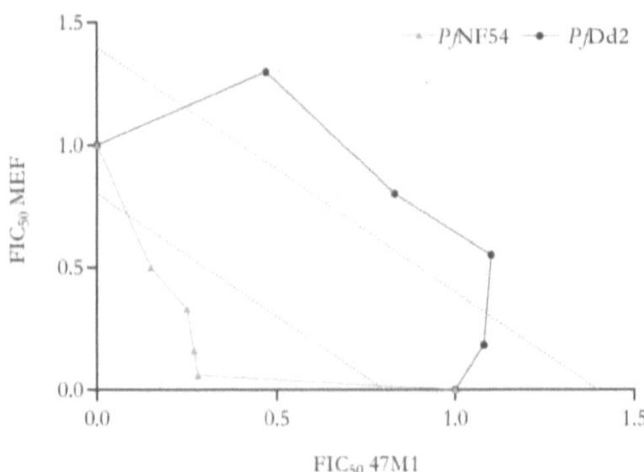

Figure 5.14. Isobologram illustrating the *in vitro* interactions of **47M1** with MEF in CQS *Pf*NF54 and CQR *Pf*Dd2 using a fixed-ratio procedure (FIC_{50} values presented as the mean, $n = 6$).

As shown in **Table 5.7** and **Table 5.8**, the overall mean ΣFIC_{50} of **43M1** or **47M1** with MEF in *Pf*NF54 was 0.64 ± 0.04 and 0.50 ± 0.07, respectively, where **47M1** displayed a greater synergistic interaction with MEF compared to **43M1** with MEF. The optimal synergistic interaction of **43M1** with MEF was achieved at the combination ratio of 1:4 of **43M1** to MEF; and for **47M1** and MEF, the greatest synergistic interaction was observed at the combination ratio of 4:1 of **47M1** to MEF.

In *Pf*Dd2, the overall antagonistic interaction of **43M1** or **47M1** with MEF was similar with an overall mean ΣFIC_{50} of 1.6 ± 0.1 for both combinations. At the combination ratios of 4:1 of **43M1** or **47M1** to MEF in *Pf*Dd2, the mean ΣFIC_{50} values were within the additive range of 0.8–1.4, however, at the higher concentrations of MEF, the interaction tended towards antagonism.

Table 5.7. *In vitro* antimalarial interactions of **43M1** with MEF against CQS *Pf*NF54 and CQR *Pf*Dd2 using a fixed-ratio isobologram method[a]

Combination ratio of 43M1:MEF	Mean ± SEM FIC$_{50}$[b]			
	*Pf*NF54		*Pf*Dd2	
	43M1	MEF	43M1	MEF
4:1	0.6 ± 0.1	0.055 ± 0.009	1.08 ± 0.07	0.11 ± 0.01
3:2	0.59 ± 0.02	0.15 ± 0.02	1.45 ± 0.09	0.40 ± 0.01
2:3	0.41 ± 0.02	0.24 ± 0.03	1.03 ± 0.03	0.641 ± 0.003
1:4	0.204 ± 0.001	0.32 ± 0.05	0.8 ± 0.2	1.0 ± 0.1
Overall mean ΣFIC$_{50}$ ± SEM	0.64 ± 0.04		1.6 ± 0.1	
Overall interaction	Synergistic		Antagonistic	

[a]IC$_{50}$ values derived using a 48 h pLDH assay. [b]n = 6.

Table 5.8. *In vitro* antimalarial interactions of **47M1** with MEF against CQS *Pf*NF54 and CQR *Pf*Dd2 using a fixed-ratio isobologram method[a]

Combination ratio of 47M1:MEF	Mean ± SEM FIC$_{50}$[b]			
	*Pf*NF54		*Pf*Dd2	
	47M1	MEF	47M1	MEF
4:1	0.28 ± 0.07	0.06 ± 0.02	1.08 ± 0.03	0.183 ± 0.06
3:2	0.27 ± 0.07	0.16 ± 0.06	1.1 ± 0.1	0.55 ± 0.09
2:3	0.25 ± 0.04	0.33 ± 0.09	0.83 ± 0.09	0.8 ± 0.1
1:4	0.15 ± 0.02	0.5 ± 0.1	0.47 ± 0.04	1.3 ± 0.2
Overall mean ΣFIC$_{50}$ ± SEM	0.50 ± 0.07		1.6 ± 0.1	
Overall interaction	Synergistic		Antagonistic	

[a]IC$_{50}$ values derived using a 48 h pLDH assay. [b]n = 6.

In CQS *Pf*NF54, **43M1** and **47M1** acted synergistically with MEF. **43M1** and **47M1** act by inhibiting haemozoin formation within the DV, which leads to a toxic build-up of FPIX.

MEF is postulated to primarily act by inhibiting protein synthesis within the parasite cytosol, and MEF has been shown to weakly inhibit haemozoin formation[77,194]. Although these drugs display seemingly unrelated primary mechanisms of action and act at different sites within the parasite, it is postulated that there is an unknown relationship between their activities which has allowed the observed enhancement in their combined antimalarial effect. This theory will require further mechanistic investigations as the data at hand is insufficient to fully explain these interactions.

In CQR *Pf*Dd2, **43M1** and **47M1** displayed an overall antagonistic interaction with MEF, especially at the higher concentration ratios of MEF to **43M1** or **47M1**. Direct or indirect interactions of MEF with the mutant drug transporter proteins of *Pf*Dd2, specifically PfCRT and possibly PfMDR1, are hypothesised to be related to the observed antagonism. In MEF-resistant strains of *P. falciparum*, PfMDR1 is responsible for transporting MEF away from its site of action, from the parasite cytosol into the DV, which alleviates its antimalarial activity[195]. Although *Pf*Dd2 does not appear to be resistant to MEF, it is speculated that MEF was able to interact with the mutant drug transporters of *Pf*Dd2 in such a way to allow the efflux of MEF into the DV; however, this process only occurs on condition that **43M1** or **47M1** is present. Subsequently, the increased concentrations of MEF in the DV could have possibly interfered with the haemozoin inhibiting activity of **43M1** and **47M1** and would, therefore, account for the antagonistic effect observed at the higher concentration ratios of MEF to the haemozoin inhibitor. MEF has been shown to bind with high affinity to FPIX, and therefore, it is plausible that MEF can demonstrate competitive binding with **43M1** or **47M1** for FPIX[228]. Furthermore, if MEF accumulated within the DV, its concentration at its primary target site within the parasite cytosol would have decreased, and this could potentially be reflected by the observed reduction in its antimalarial activity[195]. Alternatively, it is theorised that the proposed interactions of MEF with the mutant PfCRT and PfMDR transporters in *Pf*Dd2 could have competitively inhibited the binding and influx of **43M1** and **47M1** to the DV, which reduced their concentration at the site of action[168,229,230,231]. In order to support these hypotheses, comprehensive experimental evidence is required. It will be most valuable to elucidate whether if, in the presence of **43M1** or **47M1**, MEF is transported into the DV in *Pf*Dd2. This can be determined by obtaining drug accumulation data for **43M1** or **47M1** in combination with MEF in *Pf*NF54 and *Pf*Dd2.

It is theorised that parasites will not develop similar mechanisms of resistance when exposed to this combination, as quinoline resistance is primarily associated with mutations in PfCRT, whereas MEF resistance is linked to mutations in PfMDR1. Nonetheless, because strain-dependent antagonism was exhibited, the combination of **43M1** or **47M1** with MEF is unfavourable, as there is the risk of reduced antimalarial efficacy.

5.3.5. Combinations with lumefantrine

Figure 5.15, **Figure 5.16**, **Table 5.9**, and **Table 5.10** present the *in vitro* antimalarial interactions of **43M1** or **47M1** in combination with LUM against CQS *Pf*NF54 and CQR *Pf*Dd2. In the CQS strain, **43M1** and **47M1** displayed a synergistic interaction with LUM, as shown by the mean FIC_{50} values which were all below the lower limit of additivity. The CQR strain was less susceptible to the synergistic effects observed in *Pf*NF54 since **43M1** or **47M1** with LUM demonstrated an indifferent interaction in *Pf*Dd2 as displayed by the mean FIC_{50} values which were within the additivity range.

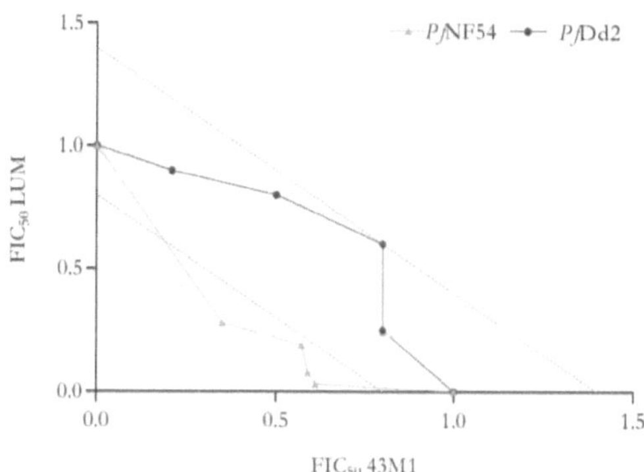

Figure 5.15. Isobologram illustrating the *in vitro* interactions of **43M1** with LUM in CQS *Pf*NF54 and CQR *Pf*Dd2 using a fixed-ratio procedure (FIC_{50} values presented as the mean, $n = 6$).

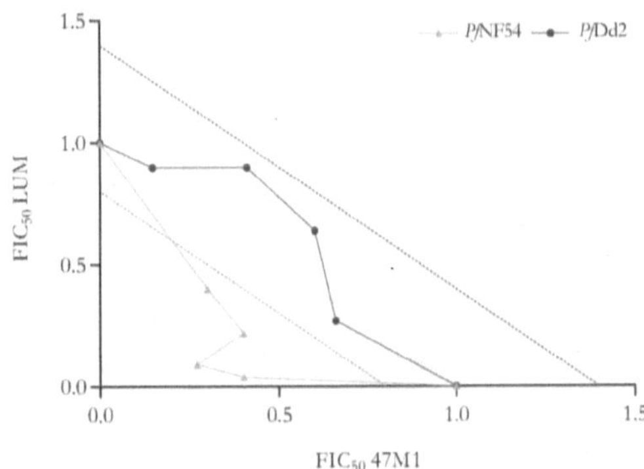

Figure 5.16. Isobologram illustrating the *in vitro* interactions of **47M1** with LUM in CQS *Pf*NF54 and CQR *Pf*Dd2 using a fixed-ratio procedure (FIC_{50} values presented as the mean, $n = 6$).

As displayed in **Table 5.9** and **Table 5.10**, the overall mean ΣFIC_{50} values of **43M1** or **47M1** with LUM in *Pf*NF54 were 0.68 ± 0.03 and 0.53 ± 0.08, respectively, which reflects a synergistic combination. However, in *Pf*Dd2, an additive interaction was demonstrated where the overall mean ΣFIC_{50} values were 1.22 ± 0.08 for **43M1** and LUM, and 1.13 ± 0.09 for **47M1** and LUM. In *Pf*NF54, all combination ratios of **43M1** with LUM displayed similar degrees of synergism, and the fixed-ratio of 3:2 of **47M1** to LUM displayed the greatest enhancement in antimalarial activity.

Table 5.9. *In vitro* antimalarial interactions of **43M1** with LUM against CQS *Pf*NF54 and CQR *Pf*Dd2 using a fixed-ratio isobologram method[a]

Combination ratio of 43M1:LUM	Mean ± SEM FIC_{50}[b]			
	*Pf*NF54		*Pf*Dd2	
	43M1	LUM	43M1	LUM
4:1	0.61 ± 0.05	0.032 ± 0.007	0.8 ± 0.1	0.25 ± 0.09
3:2	0.59 ± 0.02	0.08 ± 0.02	0.8 ± 0.1	0.6 ± 0.2
2:3	0.571 ± 0.005	0.19 ± 0.05	0.5 ± 0.2	0.8 ± 0.2
1:4	0.35 ± 0.08	0.28 ± 0.02	0.21 ± 0.07	0.9 ± 0.2
Overall mean ΣFIC_{50} ± SEM	0.68 ± 0.03		1.22 ± 0.08	
Overall interaction	Synergistic		Additive	

[a]IC_{50} values derived using a 48 h pLDH assay. [b]$n = 6$.

Table 5.10. *In vitro* antimalarial interactions of **47M1** with LUM against CQS *Pf*NF54 and CQR *Pf*Dd2 using a fixed-ratio isobologram method[a]

Combination ratio of 47M1:LUM	Mean ± SEM FIC_{50}[b]			
	*Pf*NF54		*Pf*Dd2	
	47M1	LUM	47M1	LUM
4:1	0.4 ± 0.2	0.04 ± 0.02	0.66 ± 0.03	0.27 ± 0.08
3:2	0.27 ± 0.07	0.09 ± 0.06	0.6 ± 0.2	0.64 ± 0.05
2:3	0.4 ± 0.2	0.22 ± 0.08	0.41 ± 0.09	0.9 ± 0.1
1:4	0.3 ± 0.2	0.4 ± 0.1	0.148 ± 0.008	0.9 ± 0.2
Overall mean ΣFIC_{50} ± SEM	0.53 ± 0.08		1.13 ± 0.09	
Overall interaction	Synergistic		Additive	

[a]IC_{50} values derived using a 48 h pLDH assay. [b]$n = 6$.

Since the primary mode of action of LUM is unknown, the underlying mechanisms for the observed synergy between **43M1** or **47M1** and LUM in *Pf*NF54 are unclear. The inconsistent interactions in the CQS and CQR strains of **43M1** or **47M1** in combination with LUM is tentatively hypothesised to be associated with the CQ resistance mechanisms of *Pf*Dd2, specifically the mutated drug transporter proteins, PfCRT and PfMDR1. Mutations harboured in PfCRT and PfMDR1 have been previously implicated in observed variations to LUM susceptibility, but in the presence of **43M1** or **47M1**, the interactions of LUM with the mutant transporter proteins is unknown[197]. It is challenging to rationally postulate the mechanisms behind the observed PD interactions as the experimental data presented here is limited, and the mechanistic knowledge of LUM is inadequate.

Further investigations into the drug accumulation of **43M1** or **47M1** in combination with LUM in *Pf*NF54 and *Pf*Dd2 should be performed to determine in which parasite compartment each drug is concentrated, as this will confer more understanding of their site and mode of action. The combination of **43M1** or **47M1** with LUM displayed positive interactions, although interstrain differences were observed. Since **43M1** or **47M1** and LUM do not share common resistance mechanisms, there is potential for their use as combination partners.

5.3.6. Combinations with methylene blue

Figure 5.17, **Figure 5.18**, **Table 5.11**, and **Table 5.12** present the *in vitro* antimalarial interactions of **43M1** or **47M1** in combination with MB in *Pf*NF54 and *Pf*Dd2. **43M1** and **47M1** displayed a predominately indifferent interaction with MB in CQS and CQR strains of *P. falciparum*, as displayed by their mean FIC_{50} values which generally did not deviate from the range of additivity. However, antagonism was demonstrated at one combination ratio of **47M1** to MB in *Pf*NF54.

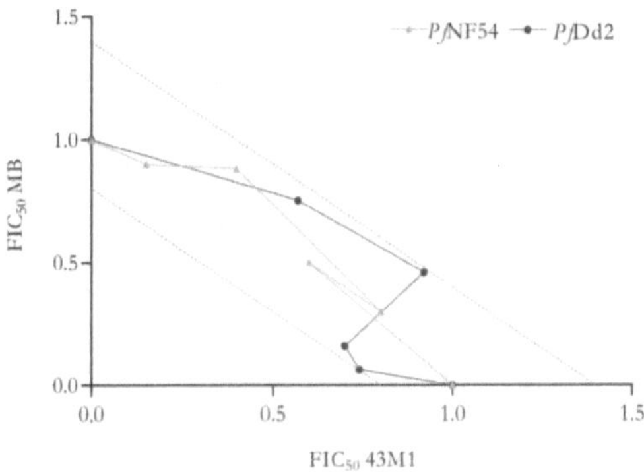

Figure 5.17. Isobologram illustrating the *in vitro* interactions of **43M1** with MB in CQS *Pf*NF54 and CQR *Pf*Dd2 using a fixed-ratio procedure (FIC_{50} values presented as the mean, $n = 6$).

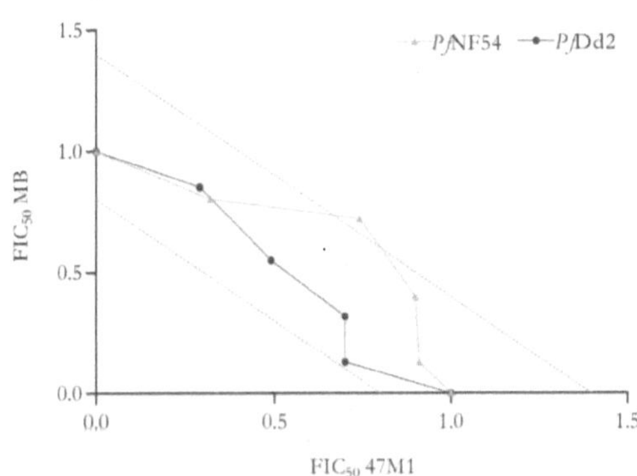

Figure 5.18. Isobologram illustrating the *in vitro* interactions of **47M1** with MB in CQS *Pf*NF54 and CQR *Pf*Dd2 using a fixed-ratio procedure (FIC_{50} values presented as the mean, $n = 6$).

The combination of **43M1** and MB displayed overall mean ΣFIC_{50} values of 1.13 ± 0.05 and 1.1 ± 0.1 in *Pf*NF54 and *Pf*Dd2, respectively. **47M1** and MB demonstrated overall mean ΣFIC_{50} values of 1.23 ± 0.09 in *Pf*NF54 and 1.01 ± 0.07 in *Pf*Dd2. Although the interaction tended towards antagonism at the concentration ratio of 2:3 of **47M1** to MB in *Pf*NF54, the predominant effect was indifferent as displayed by the overall ΣFIC_{50} value, which was within the range of additivity.

Table 5.11. *In vitro* antimalarial interactions of **43M1** with MB against CQS *Pf*NF54 and CQR *Pf*Dd2 using a fixed-ratio isobologram method[a]

Combination ratio of 43M1:MB	Mean ± SEM FIC_{50}[b]			
	*Pf*NF54		*Pf*Dd2	
	43M1	**MB**	**43M1**	**MB**
4:1	0.6 ± 0.2	0.5 ± 0.3	0.74 ± 0.09	0.063 ± 0.005
3:2	0.8 ± 0.2	0.3 ± 0.1	0.7 ± 0.1	0.16 ± 0.02
2:3	0.4 ± 0.2	0.88 ± 0.03	0.92 ± 0.07	0.46 ± 0.06
1:4	0.15 ± 0.05	0.9 ± 0.1	0.57 ± 0.03	0.75 ± 0.08
Overall mean ΣFIC_{50} ± SEM	1.13 ± 0.05		1.1 ± 0.1	
Overall interaction	Additive		Additive	

[a]IC_{50} values derived using a 48 h pLDH assay. [b]$n = 6$.

Table 5.12. *In vitro* antimalarial interactions of **47M1** with MB against CQS *Pf*NF54 and CQR *Pf*Dd2 using a fixed-ratio isobologram method[a]

Combination ratio of 47M1:MB	Mean ± SEM FIC_{50}[b]			
	*Pf*NF54		*Pf*Dd2	
	47M1	**MB**	**47M1**	**MB**
4:1	0.91 ± 0.03	0.13 ± 0.02	0.7 ± 0.1	0.130 ± 0.007
3:2	0.9 ± 0.4	0.4 ± 0.2	0.7 ± 0.1	0.32 ± 0.01
2:3	0.74 ± 0.05	0.72 ± 0.06	0.49 ± 0.06	0.55 ± 0.04
1:4	0.32 ± 0.07	0.8 ± 0.2	0.29 ± 0.05	0.85 ± 0.02
Overall mean ΣFIC_{50} ± SEM	1.23 ± 0.09		1.01 ± 0.07	
Overall interaction	Additive		Additive	

[a]IC_{50} values derived using a 48 h pLDH assay. [b]$n = 6$.

The overall degree of additivity between **43M1** or **47M1** and MB was similar in *Pf*NF54 and *Pf*Dd2, which suggests that the CQ resistance mechanisms did not have a significant effect on their interactions. MB has been shown to interfere with the redox balance within the parasite by specifically inhibiting GR; and the PDBQ compounds target the FPIX crystallisation pathway. It is postulated that the observed additive interaction is reflective of the differences in the target sites of MB and the PDBQ metabolites, and, furthermore, the differences in their stage specificity. MB has been shown to act predominately on ring-stage and early trophozoite-stage parasites, whereas **43M1** and **47M1** are hypothesised to act primarily during the trophozoite stage, therefore, it is plausible that each antimalarial acted independently from one another at different stages of the lifecycle[77,202]. The stage specificity of each drug in combination will need to be determined to support this conjecture.

Although **43M1** or **47M1** with MB did not potentiate antimalarial activity, they can still be considered as potential combination partners. However, further knowledge of their mechanistic action will be needed to determine if there is a possibility that this combination will develop similar mechanisms of resistance.

5.3.7. Combinations with atovaquone

Figure 5.19, **Figure 5.20**, **Table 5.13**, and **Table 5.14** present the *in vitro* antimalarial interactions of **43M1** or **47M1** in combination with ATOV against CQS *Pf*NF54 and CQR *Pf*Dd2. The isobolograms illustrate synergistic interactions which were consistent in both the CQS and CQR strains as shown by the mean FIC_{50} values, which were predominately below the lower limit of additivity. For both combinations in *Pf*NF54, an additive interaction was observed for one of the three fixed-dose ratios, as displayed by the mean FIC_{50} value which was above the lower limit of additivity.

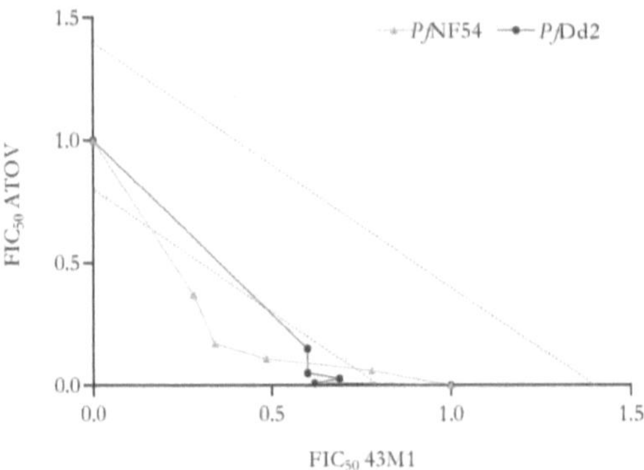

Figure 5.19. Isobologram illustrating the *in vitro* interactions of **43M1** with ATOV in CQS *Pf*NF54 and CQR *Pf*Dd2 using a fixed-ratio procedure (FIC_{50} values presented as the mean, $n = 6$).

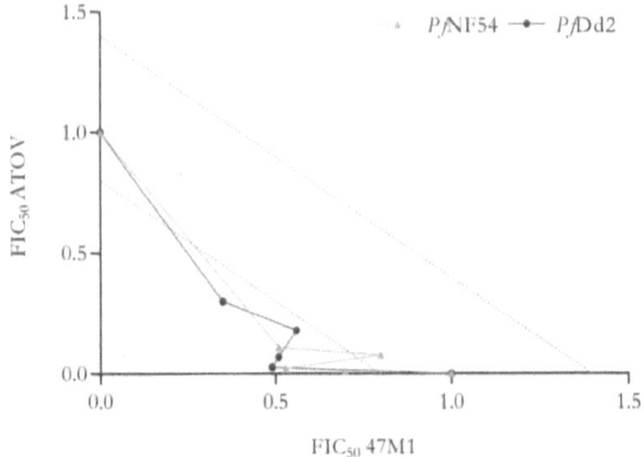

Figure 5.20. Isobologram illustrating the *in vitro* interactions of **47M1** with ATOV in CQS *Pf*NF54 and CQR *Pf*Dd2 using a fixed-ratio procedure (FIC_{50} values presented as the mean, $n = 6$).

Although there were variations in the interactions between **43M1** or **47M1** with ATOV in *Pf*NF54, the overall interactions were synergistic as displayed by the mean overall ΣFIC_{50} values. **43M1** and ATOV displayed overall synergistic interactions of 0.65 ± 0.07 in *Pf*NF54 and 0.69 ± 0.03 in *Pf*Dd2; and **47M1** and ATOV demonstrated similar synergistic interactions with overall ΣFIC_{50} values of 0.69 ± 0.07 and 0.62 ± 0.05 in *Pf*NF54 and *Pf*Dd2, respectively. The additive interactions in *Pf*NF54 were exhibited at the combination ratios of 4:1 of **43M1** to ATOV and 2:3 of **47M1** to ATOV.

Table 5.13. *In vitro* antimalarial interactions of **43M1** with ATOV against CQS *Pf*NF54 and CQR *Pf*Dd2 using a fixed-ratio isobologram method[a]

Combination ratio of 43M1:ATOV	Mean ± SEM FIC_{50}[b]			
	*Pf*NF54		*Pf*Dd2	
	43M1	ATOV	43M1	ATOV
4:1	0.78 ± 0.06	0.06 ± 0.02	0.62 ± 0.01	0.009 ± 0.001
3:2	0.49 ± 0.03	0.11 ± 0.02	0.69 ± 0.01	0.028 ± 0.002
2:3	0.34 ± 0.06	0.17 ± 0.01	0.6 ± 0.2	0.05 ± 0.01
1:4	0.28 ± 0.04	0.37 ± 0.04	0.6 ± 0.1	0.15 ± 0.02
Overall mean ΣFIC_{50} ± SEM	0.65 ± 0.07		0.69 ± 0.03	
Overall interaction	Synergistic		Synergistic	

[a]IC_{50} values derived using a 48 h pLDH assay. [b]n = 6.

Table 5.14. *In vitro* antimalarial interactions of **47M1** with ATOV against CQS *Pf*NF54 and CQR *Pf*Dd2 using a fixed-ratio isobologram method[a]

Combination ratio of 47M1:ATOV	Mean ± SEM FIC_{50}[b]			
	*Pf*NF54		*Pf*Dd2	
	47M1	ATOV	47M1	ATOV
4:1	0.698 ± 0.002	0.014 ± 0.004	0.49 ± 0.03	0.03 ± 0.02
3:2	0.53 ± 0.07	0.024 ± 0.004	0.51 ± 0.09	0.07 ± 0.03
2:3	0.8 ± 0.1	0.078 ± 0.008	0.56 ± 0.08	0.18 ± 0.08
1:4	0.51 ± 0.01	0.111 ± 0.001	0.35 ± 0.08	0.3 ± 0.1
Overall mean ΣFIC_{50} ± SEM	0.69 ± 0.07		0.62 ± 0.05	
Overall interaction	Synergistic		Synergistic	

[a]IC_{50} values derived using a 48 h pLDH assay. [b]n = 6.

The overall degree of synergy between **43M1** or **47M1** and ATOV was similar in *Pf*NF54 and *Pf*Dd2, which suggests that the CQ resistance mechanisms did not affect the interactions. The PDBQ metabolites act by inhibiting the FPIX crystallisation pathway within the DV, and ATOV targets the cytochrome bc_1 complex, which is involved with the electron transport system within the mitochondria[77,208]. The unique mechanisms of action and the distinct target sites of **43M1** or **47M1** and ATOV would predict an indifferent interaction; however, as observed, there was potentiation in antimalarial activity when used in combination. This could reflect an unknown cooperative role in the action of **43M1** or **47M1** and ATOV.

At the higher concentration ratios of 4:1 and 3:2 of **43M1** or **47M1** to ATOV, the activity of ATOV was greatly enhanced as displayed by the mean FIC_{50} values of ATOV in *Pf*NF54 and *Pf*Dd2 which ranged from 0.009 ± 0.001 to 0.11 ± 0.02 for **43M1** and ATOV, and from 0.014 ± 0.004 to 0.07 ± 0.03 for **47M1** and ATOV. This suggests that **43M1** and **47M1** were able to potentiate the antimalarial activity of ATOV through some unknown mechanism. Therefore, **43M1** or **47M1** with ATOV revealed promising *in vitro* interactions, in addition to displaying distinct modes of action, this combination was able to augment antimalarial activity.

5.3.8. Study limitations

The nature of the interactions of the drug combinations were determined using a 48 h incubation which encompassed one lifecycle; therefore, the inhibitory effects of drugs which act at a later stage in the lifecycle might not be accurately captured. Additionally, a longer treatment time could enhance the overall inhibitory effect and provide a more accurate representation of the interaction, especially for drugs which display a delayed onset of activity or unknown mechanism of action. Additionally, further knowledge into the genetic background conferring CQ resistance in *Pf*Dd2 is needed as this was a common limitation when discussing the observed interactions in this strain.

5.4. CONCLUSION

Given the use of combination therapy in delaying the emergence of drug resistance, a preliminary evaluation of the *in vitro* interactions of **43M1** and **47M1** with clinically relevant antimalarials was explored to elucidate potential combination partners, with different mechanisms of action, that can be prioritised for further development. The findings from this study revealed favourable synergistic *in vitro* interactions of **43M1** or **47M1** with DHA or ATOV in *Pf*NF54 and *Pf*Dd2, which demonstrates their prospective use in combination therapy. Additionally, by exploiting their observed synergy, these combinations could potentially reflect enhanced antimalarial potency. Further investigations into the *in vivo* interactions and antimalarial efficacy of these combinations are warranted as PK differences may alter the observed *in vitro* drug interactions. Lastly, from the data presented in this isobologram study, **43M1** and **47M1** were unable to reverse CQ resistance; this suggests that the combination of **43M1** or **47M1** with CQ should not be further investigated to fulfil the intention of targeting CQR strains.

CHAPTER VI

CONCLUSIONS AND FUTURE STUDIES

6. CONCLUSIONS AND FUTURE STUDIES

6.1. Conclusions

Given the persistent challenge of antimalarial drug resistance, continued investment towards drug discovery and development programs is essential for effective disease management. Reports of the current frontline ART-based treatment displaying reduced clinical efficacy has highlighted the necessity for alternative therapies[17].

To address this need, a novel series of PDBQ compounds were designed to chemosensitise CQR strains of *P. falciparum*. Although these compounds displayed promising *in vitro* antiplasmodial activity, they were shown to be metabolically labile. A metabolite identification study revealed that the major metabolites retained the antiplasmodial pharmacophore of the parent PDBQ compound. The pre-synthesised major metabolites displayed promising *in vitro* activity through the inhibition of haemozoin formation resulting in a toxic accumulation of FPIX. Additionally, these metabolic derivatives displayed favourable *in vitro* ADME properties[75,77]. Consequently, the promising *in vitro* characteristics of the PDBQ series of metabolites initiated their further development.

In this study, the major metabolites of the PDBQ parent compounds were evaluated to identify potential preclinical antimalarial lead candidates. Rational lead selection was guided by determining the *in vivo* PK of the parent compounds and major metabolites in a healthy murine model. Compounds that exhibited favourable PK profiles progressed to the next phase of the study which evaluated the *in vivo* antimalarial efficacy and the PK/PD relationship of the lead compounds in a *P. falciparum Pf*3D7-infected humanised murine model.

Prior to the PK studies, bioanalytical methods were developed for the quantitative analysis of the PDBQ parent compounds and major metabolites in whole blood. Given the early phase of this preclinical study, the HPLC-MS/MS assays were partially validated based on a fit-for-purpose approach with assessed assay sensitivity, selectivity, accuracy, precision, matrix effects, and analyte stability through various experimental procedures. This ensured that the generated PK concentration data was accurate and reliable.

Lastly, the potential of the lead candidates to be used in combination therapy with established antimalarials and the ability of the lead candidates to reverse CQR was investigated using fixed-dose ratio isobologram analyses.

In addition to the *in vitro* antiplasmodial activity, selectivity, cytotoxicity, and ADME, compound progression was also directed by the *in vivo* PK properties; as the concentration of the drug at the site of action governs the antimalarial response, where a higher concentration translates to a greater therapeutic effect[118]. The PK analyses in healthy mice revealed that the C_{max} and exposure of the antimalarial pharmacophore were greater after direct oral administration of the preformed metabolite compared to the cumulative C_{max} and exposure of the parent and formed metabolites after administration of the parent compound. Therefore, the parent compound was not used to deliver the major metabolites, but rather, the pre-synthesised active metabolite was directly administered.

Table 6.1 presents a comparative summary of the *in vitro* antiplasmodial activity and the oral PK parameters in healthy mice of the PDBQ parent compounds and major metabolites. **43M1** and **47M1** demonstrated their ability to reach and sustain relatively high concentrations with C_{max} and $AUC_{0-\infty}$ values of 8 ± 1 μM and 62 ± 3 μM.h, respectively for **43M1** and 9.4 ± 0.5 μM and 93 ± 9 μM.h, respectively for **47M1**. Furthermore, **43M1** and **47M1** maintained therapeutic levels which exceeded each compound's respective *in vitro* *Pf*3D7 IC_{50} at 24 h post-oral administration by 10.5- and 57.9-fold for **43M1** and **47M1**, respectively. These observations were hypothesised to translate to efficacious *in vivo* antimalarial activity and, therefore, **43M1** and **47M1** were evaluated for their ability to suppress parasite proliferation in a *P. falciparum*-infected murine model.

Table 6.1. Summary of the *in vitro* antiplasmodial activities and the *in vivo* non-compartmental PK parameters in healthy mice of the PDBQ parent compounds and their major metabolites[77]

Experimental compound	***In vitro* IC$_{50}$ (μM)**		***In vivo* PK parameter after a 20 mg/kg oral administration of the experimental compound**			
	***Pf*3D7**	***Pf*Dd2**	**Analyte**	**C$_{max}$ (μM)**	**AUC$_{0-\infty}$ (μM.h)**	**F (%)**
49	0.061	0.137	**49**	0.22 ± 0.04	1.1 ± 0.1	2.2
			49M1	0.6 ± 0.1	3.1 ± 0.3	-
			49M2	1.1 ± 0.1	6.7 ± 0.3	-
49M1	0.009	0.051	**49M1**	2.4 ± 0.3	16 ± 2	22.2
49M2	0.019	0.063	**49M2**	6.0 ± 0.5	28 ± 1	28.1
43	0.038	0.124	**43**	0.32 ± 0.04	1.3 ± 0.3	7.5
			43M1	0.50 ± 0.03	4.4 ± 0.9	-
			43M2	0.31 ± 0.05	3 ± 1	-
43M1	0.016	0.078	**43M1**	8 ± 1	62 ± 3	42.3
43M2	0.036	0.255	**43M2**	8.5 ± 0.5	51 ± 2	25.1
47	0.033	0.151	**47**	1.09 ± 0.03	3.93 ± 0.05	24.6
			47M1	0.54 ± 0.07	8.4 ± 0.4	-
			47M2	0.23 ± 0.02	3.3 ± 0.1	-
47M1	0.013	0.055	**47M1**	9.4 ± 0.5	93 ± 9	42.0

In a *P. falciparum*-infected NSG murine model, **43M1** and **47M1** exhibited a 98% reduction in parasitaemia after four daily consecutive oral administrations of 20 mg/kg of **43M1** or **47M1** compared to the untreated control. As presented in **Table 6.2**, the concentration-effect relationship, as described by the $C_{maxED90}$ and AUC_{ED90}, showed that **47M1** displayed a relatively higher maximal concentration and oral exposure at the ED_{90} compared to **43M1**, this likely attributed to the 1.5-fold lower observed ED_{90} for **47M1** compared to **43M1**. In addition, flow cytometry dot plots, illustrating the changes in the morphological subpopulations after treatment with **43M1** or **47M1**, suggests that the compounds cleared or arrested the development of trophozoite-stage parasites which ultimately hindered parasite proliferation. This observation correlates to the proposed stage specificity of **43M1** and **47M1** as these haemozoin-inhibiting compounds are hypothesised to act on trophozoite-stage parasites which are actively catabolising haemoglobin.

Table 6.2. Summary of the PK/PD parameters of **43M1** and **47M1** in a *P. falciparum*-infected NSG murine model

PK/PD parameter	43M1	47M1
ED_{90} (mg/kg)	12	7.7
$C_{maxED90}$ (μM)	0.81	1.2
AUC_{ED90} (μM.h)	6.2	18.6

Lastly, given the significance of combination therapy in delaying the emergence of drug resistance, the potential of **43M1** and **47M1** to be used as a partner drug was explored. The *in vitro* combination studies, using isobologram analyses, evaluated the interactions of **43M1** or **47M1** with established antimalarials, which exhibit mechanisms of action unrelated to haemozoin inhibition; as this approach is expected to reduce the drug selective pressure.

As displayed in **Table 6.3**, **43M1** and **47M1** were synergistic with DHA or ATOV and additive with MB in a CQS and CQR strain of *P. falciparum*. **43M1** and **47M1** were synergistic with MEF or LUM in a CQS strain of *P. falciparum*; however, the combinations with MEF or LUM in the CQR strain of *P. falciparum* displayed antagonism and additivity, respectively. Additionally, since a portion of the proposed CQ-resistance reversing dibenzylmethylamine side chain of the parent compound is cleaved off to produce the PDBQ metabolites, it was unknown whether **43M1** and **47M1** interacted with the CQR PfCRT in a manner which chemosensitises CQR parasites. Therefore, the ability of the lead candidates, and their parent PDBQ compound, to reverse CQ resistance was evaluated in a CQR strain of *P. falciparum*. The parent PDBQ compounds, **43** and **47**, displayed synergy with CQ in CQR *P. falciparum*, however, **43M1** and **47M1** exhibited additive interactions with CQ and were unable to potentiate the antiplasmodial activity of CQ in the CQR strain. This should not pose a setback to the developability of the lead metabolite candidates as pertinently, they were still favourably active in a CQR strain of *P. falciparum* and they, therefore, do not share cross-resistance with CQ.

Priority should be given to combination partners possessing distinct mechanisms of action to haemozoin inhibition, as they are likely to display dissimilar mechanisms of resistance. Therefore, reflecting on the original concept of the PDBQ compounds, although **43M1** and **47M1** do not appear to reverse CQ resistance, they still displayed promising synergistic interactions with DHA and ATOV in CQS and CQR strains of *P. falciparum* which, therefore, merits further progression of **43M1** and **47M1** where a greater focus should be placed on developing these compounds as a partner drug in combination therapy.

Table 6.3. Summary of the overall *in vitro* interactions of **43M1** or **47M1** with clinically relevant antimalarials in CQS *Pf*NF54 and CQR *Pf*Dd2 using a fixed-dose ratio isobologram procedure

Partner drug	43M1		47M1	
	*Pf*NF54	*Pf*Dd2	*Pf*NF54	*Pf*Dd2
CQ	-[a]	Additivity	-[a]	Additivity
DHA	Synergy	Synergy	Synergy	Synergy
MEF	Synergy	Antagonism	Synergy	Antagonism
LUM	Synergy	Additivity	Synergy	Additivity
MB	Additivity	Additivity	Additivity	Additivity
ATOV	Synergy	Synergy	Synergy	Synergy

[a]Not determined.

6.2. Future studies

Given the early stage of this preclinical evaluation, there still remain numerous unknown *in vitro* and *in vivo* properties of **43M1** and **47M1**, which should be explored to expand on the existing knowledge of the lead candidates. This will provide understanding into whether **43M1** or **47M1** exhibit properties that make them superior to other haemozoin-inhibiting compounds which are currently in various phases of preclinical or clinical development. These insights will subsequently guide future decisions as to whether **43M1** or **47M1** should progress to the next phase in the drug-development pipeline.

The following summarises proposed future work stemming directly from the results presented in this study;

i. As discussed in **Chapter IV**, addressing batch to batch variation in the synthesis of the PDBQ compound, as this could alter compound solubility as well as the observed antiplasmodial activity. *In vitro* assays which determine the solubility in biorelevant media should be performed to ensure relatively consistent pharmacological and ADME properties between synthesised batches[232].

ii. As discussed in **Chapter III** and **Chapter IV**, investigating the degree of PPB in relevant matrices, such as in murine plasma and humanised murine plasma, using, for example, ultracentrifugation techniques[233]. This evaluation can be performed to determine the unbound drug concentrations obtained from the *in vivo* PK experiments in healthy and malaria-infected mice, as this will provide a more accurate reflection of the free drug which is available to exert the pharmacological effect. Additionally, the corrected free fraction of the maximal concentration will provide a more accurate reflection of the toxicity liabilities of the PDBQ compounds.

iii. As discussed in **Chapter IV**, investigating the degree of accumulation of **43M1** or **47M1** in malaria-infected and uninfected erythrocytes[234]. In addition to the PPB data, these parameters will provide valuable information which can aid in further interpreting the data from the *in vivo* PK experiments in healthy and malaria-infected mice. Furthermore, as discussed in **Chapter V**, the degree of accumulation and distribution of **43M1** or **47M1** alone, and in combination with a selected partner drug, should be explored in different parasite organelles[235]. This will assist in understanding the underlying mechanisms of the interactions presented in the *in vitro* antimalarial combination studies.

The following proposes recommendations for other future work which can be explored to broaden the preclinical characterisation of the lead PDBQ candidates;

i. To further explore the *in vitro* antiplasmodial activities, **43M1** and **47M1** should be tested against a wider panel of *P. falciparum* clinical isolates, including strains which display resistance towards clinically employed antimalarials. This will elucidate any compromising existence of cross-resistance, especially against proposed partner drugs; and could possibly provide insights into the unknown resistance mechanisms of **43M1** and **47M1**, which is hypothesised to be related to DV membrane transport proteins, as previously demonstrated with CQ[61]. Although **43M1** and **47M1** have exhibited activity against asexual intraerythrocytic *P. falciparum*, it will be valuable to investigate whether they are possibly active during the liver and sexual gametocyte stages of the parasite lifecycle. Gametocytocidal activity can be determined by means of membrane feeding assays which assess transmission-blocking potential[236]. Hepatic activity can be assessed using an *in vitro* assay which determines the inhibitory effect on parasites infected in HepG2 cells, a human liver cancer cell line[237]. Lastly, the proclivity of parasites to develop resistance towards the lead PDBQ compounds should be determined using *in vitro* drug pressure assays which select for resistant strains and assess the liability of the *in vitro* rate of the emergence of drug resistance[238,239]. Together these studies could reveal possible alternative mechanisms of action to haemozoin inhibition.

ii. To further address compound safety, a series of *in vitro* assays should be performed to establish the risks associated with cytotoxicity, genotoxicity and importantly, hERG toxicity which commonly manifests in quinoline-containing drugs[76]. **43M1** and **47M1** displayed minimal toxicity against the CHO cell line; however, it will be valuable to further characterise their toxicity against other standard mammalian cell lines, such as Vero cells which are derived from the kidney of an African green monkey[240]. The potential of **43M1** and **47M1** to damage genetic material can be determined using the Ames test which examines the genotoxic effect of a compound in a bacterial strain, *Salmonella typhimurium*[241]. The hERG liability can be assessed using electrophysiological patch clamp assays which determine compound interactions with the hERG ion channel[242]. Additionally, a CYP inhibition assay can be performed to assess the possibility of drug-drug interactions which could lead to adverse drug reactions[243]. Lastly, the potential risk of **43M1** and **47M1** in patients with glucose-6-phosphate dehydrogenase, or G6PD, deficiency should be determined early during the preclinical development phase as drug-induced haemolysis related to G6PD deficiency has been commonly reported during antimalarial therapy[244].

iii. To further investigate the *in vivo* antimalarial efficacy of **43M1** and **47M1** in an NSG murine model infected with a CQR strain of *P. falciparum*[153]. **43M1** and **47M1** displayed *in vitro* IC_{50} values in CQR *Pf*Dd2 which were 4.9- and 4.2-fold higher, respectively than their *in vitro* activities in CQS *Pf*3D7; and it is unknown whether these differences in activity are significant enough to limit their *in vivo* efficacy. Additionally, dose fractionation studies for **43M1** and **47M1** can be performed to further elucidate the PK/PD relationship by determining the concentration- or time-dependent PK drivers of efficacy, as this will aid in rational dose selection for future studies[144]. Lastly, the *in vivo* PK and antimalarial efficacy of **43M1** or **47M1** and the selected partner drug should be evaluated in a malaria-infected murine model to determine the combination potential in a system which takes into account the PK differences of each drug, specifically related to differences in the $T_{1/2}$, Cl, and V_d.

In conclusion, the study presented in this thesis selected two antimalarial lead candidates, from the series of PDBQ parents and major metabolites, which demonstrated efficacy in a *P. falciparum*-infected NSG murine model. Additionally, the potential of the lead candidates to be used as a synergistic partner drug in combination therapy was demonstrated using *in vitro* antimalarial isobologram analyses. Further development of **43M1** and **47M1** is warranted; but, their continued progress should be supported by investigations which highlight their advantages over prevailing preclinical and clinical antimalarials which exhibit comparable mechanisms of action.

CHAPTER VII

REFERENCES

1. World Malaria Report 2019. (World Health Organisation, Geneva, 2019).

2. Greenwood, B. M., Bojang, K., Whitty, C. J. M. & Targett, G. A. T. Malaria. *The Lancet* **365**, 1487-1498 (2005).

3. Miller, R. L. *et al.* Diagnosis of *Plasmodium falciparum* Infections in Mummies using the Rapid Manual ParaSight™-F test. *Transactions of The Royal Society of Tropical Medicine and Hygiene* **88**, 31-32 (1994).

4. Cox, F. E. G. History of Human Parasitology. *Clinical Microbiology Reviews* **15**, 595-612 (2002).

5. Hempelmann, E. & Krafts, K. Bad Air, Amulets and Mosquitoes: 2,000 Years of Changing Perspectives on Malaria. *Malaria Journal* **12**, 232-232 (2013).

6. Laveran, A. Note sur un Nouveau Parasite Trouvé dans le Sang de Plusieurs Malades Atteints de Fièvre Palustre. *Bulletin de l'Academie Medicale* **9**, 1235-1236 (1880).

7. Ross, R. *Memoirs with a Full Account of the Great Malaria Problem and its Solution.* (1923).

8. Manson, P. Experimental Proof of the Mosquito-Malaria Theory. *British Medical Journal* **2**, 949 (1900).

9. Achan, J. *et al.* Quinine, an Old Anti-Malarial Drug in a Modern World: Role in the Treatment of Malaria. *Malaria Journal* **10**, 144 (2011).

10. Coatney, G. R. Pitfalls in a Discovery: The Chronicle of Chloroquine. *The American Journal of Tropical Medicine and Hygiene* **12**, 121-128 (1963).

11. Peters, W. *Chemotherapy and Drug Resistance in Malaria 2nd ed.* (Academic Press, 1987).

12. Cowman, A. F. & Foote, S. J. Chemotherapy and Drug Resistance in Malaria. *International Journal for Parasitology* **20**, 503-513 (1990).

13. Klayman, D. Qinghaosu (Artemisinin): An Antimalarial Drug from China. *Science* **228**, 1049-1055 (1985).

14. Arrow, K. J., Panosian, C. & Gelband, H. The Human and Economic Burden of Malaria. in *Saving Lives, Buying Time: Economics of Malaria Drugs in an Age of Resistance* 168-196 (The National Academies Press, 2004).

15. Eastman, R. T. & Fidock, D. A. Artemisinin-Based Combination Therapies: A Vital Tool in Efforts to Eliminate Malaria. *Nature Reviews Microbiology* **7**, 864-874 (2009).

16. White, N. Delaying Antimalarial Drug Resistance with Combination Chemotherapy. *Parassitologia* **41**, 301-308 (1999).

17. Dondorp, A. M. *et al.* Artemisinin Resistance in *Plasmodium falciparum* Malaria. *New England Journal of Medicine* **361**, 455-467 (2009).

18. Noedl, H. *et al.* Evidence of Artemisinin-Resistant Malaria in Western Cambodia. *New England Journal of Medicine* **359**, 2619-2620 (2008).

19. Burrows, J. N. *et al.* New Developments in Anti-Malarial Target Candidate and Product Profiles. *Malaria Journal* **16**, 26 (2017).

20. Wells, T. N. C., van Huijsduijnen, R. H. & Van Voorhis, W. C. Malaria Medicines: A Glass Half Full? *Nature Reviews Drug Discovery* **14**, 424-442 (2015).

21. Efficacy and Safety of RTS,S/AS01 Malaria Vaccine with or without a Booster Dose in Infants and Children in Africa: Final Results of a Phase 3, Individually Randomised, Controlled Trial. *The Lancet* **386**, 31-45 (2015).

22. Hill, A. V. S. Vaccines Against Malaria. *Philosophical Transactions of the Royal Society B: Biological Sciences* **366**, 2806-2814 (2011).

23. Francis, S. E., Sullivan, J., D.J. & Goldberg, D. E. Hemoglobin Metabolism in the Malaria Parasite *Plasmodium falciparum*. *Annual Review of Microbiology* **51**, 97-123 (1997).

24. Aly, A. S. I., Vaughan, A. M. & Kappe, S. H. I. Malaria Parasite Development in the Mosquito and Infection of the Mammalian Host. *Annual Review of Microbiology* **63**, 195-221 (2009).

25. Baton, L. A. & Ranford-Cartwright, L. C. Spreading the Seeds of Million-Murdering Death: Metamorphoses of Malaria in the Mosquito. *Trends in Parasitology* **21**, 573-580 (2005).

26. Maier, A., Matuschewski, K., Zhang, M. & Rug, M. *Plasmodium falciparum*. *Trends in Parasitology* **35**, 481-482 (2019).

27. Siciliano, G. & Alano, P. Enlightening the Malaria Parasite Life Cycle: Bioluminescent *Plasmodium* in Fundamental and Applied Research. *Frontiers in Microbiology* **6** (2015).

28. Krugliak, M., Zhang, J. & Ginsburg, H. Intraerythrocytic *Plasmodium falciparum* Utilizes Only a Fraction of the Amino Acids Derived from the Digestion of Host Cell Cytosol for the Biosynthesis of its Proteins. *Molecular and Biochemical Parasitology* **119**, 249-256 (2002).

29. Ginsburg, H., Famin, O., Zhang, J. & Krugliak, M. Inhibition of Glutathione-Dependent Degradation of Heme by Chloroquine and Amodiaquine as a Possible Basis for their Antimalarial Mode of Action. *Biochemical Pharmacology* **56**, 1305-1313 (1998).

30. Yayon, A., Waa, J. A. V., Yayon, M., Geary, T. G. & Jensen, J. B. Stage-Dependent Effects of Chloroquine on *Plasmodium falciparum In Vitro*. *The Journal of Protozoology* **30**, 642-647 (1983).

31. Langreth, S. G., Jensen, J. B., Reese, R. T. & Trager, W. Fine Structure of Human Malaria *In Vitro*. *The Journal of Protozoology* **25**, 443-452 (1978).

32. Slomianny, C. Three-Dimensional Reconstruction of the Feeding Process of the Malaria Parasite. *Blood Cells* **16**, 369-378 (1990).

33. Olliaro, P. & Goldberg, D. The *Plasmodium* Digestive Vacuole: Metabolic Headquarters and Choice Drug Target. *Parasitology Today* **11**, 294-297 (1995).

34. Yayon, A., Cabantchik, Z. & Ginsburg, H. Identification of the Acidic Compartment of *Plasmodium falciparum*-Infected Human Erythrocytes as the Target of the Antimalarial Drug Chloroquine. *The EMBO Journal* **3**, 2695-2700 (1984).

35. Fairfield, A. S., Abosch, A., Ranz, A., Eaton, J. W. & Meshnick, S. R. Oxidant Defense Enzymes of *Plasmodium falciparum*. *Molecular and Biochemical Parasitology* **30**, 77-82 (1988).

36. Chou, A. C. & Fitch, C. D. Mechanism of Hemolysis Induced by Ferriprotoporphyrin IX. *The Journal of Clinical Investigation* **68**, 672-677 (1981).

37. Fitch, C. D. *et al.* Lysis of *Plasmodium falciparum* by Ferriprotoporphyrin IX and a Chloroquine-Ferriprotoporphyrin IX Complex. *Antimicrobial Agents and Chemotherapy* **21**, 819-822 (1982).

38. Schmitt, T. H., Frezzatti, W. A. & Schreier, S. Hemin-Induced Lipid Membrane Disorder and Increased Permeability: A Molecular Model for the Mechanism of Cell Lysis. *Archives of Biochemistry and Biophysics* **307**, 96-103 (1993).

39. Brown, W. Malarial Pigment (So-Called Melanin): Its Nature and Mode of Production. *The Journal of Experimental Medicine* **13**, 290-299 (1911).

40. Pagola, S., Stephens, P. W., Bohle, D. S., Kosar, A. D. & Madsen, S. K. The Structure of Malaria Pigment β-Haematin. *Nature* **404**, 307-310 (2000).

41. Egan, T. J. *et al.* Fate of Haem Iron in the Malaria Parasite *Plasmodium falciparum*. *Biochemical Journal* **365**, 343-347 (2002).

42. Gildenhuys, J., Roex, T. l., Egan, T. J. & de Villiers, K. A. The Single Crystal X-ray Structure of β-Hematin DMSO Solvate Grown in the Presence of Chloroquine, a β-Hematin Growth-Rate Inhibitor. *Journal of the American Chemical Society* **135**, 1037-1047 (2013).

43. Slater, A. F. *et al.* An Iron-Carboxylate Bond Links the Heme Units of Malaria Pigment. *Proceedings of the National Academy of Sciences of the United States of America* **88**, 325-329 (1991).

44. Cohen, S. N., Phifer, K. O. & Yielding, K. L. Complex Formation between Chloroquine and Ferrihæmic Acid In Vitro, and its Effect on the Antimalarial Action of Chloroquine. *Nature* **202**, 805-806 (1964).

45. Chou, A. C., Chevli, R. & Fitch, C. D. Ferriprotoporphyrin IX Fulfills the Criteria for Identification as the Chloroquine Receptor of Malaria Parasites. *Biochemistry* **19**, 1543-1549 (1980).

46. Sullivan, D. J., Gluzman, I. Y., Russell, D. G. & Goldberg, D. E. On the Molecular Mechanism of Chloroquine's Antimalarial Action. *Proceedings of the National Academy of Sciences* **93**, 11865-11870 (1996).

47. Dorn, A. *et al.* An Assessment of Drug-Haematin Binding as a Mechanism for Inhibition of Haematin Polymerisation by Quinoline Antimalarials. *Biochemical Pharmacology* **55**, 727-736 (1998).

48. Buller, R., Peterson, M. L., Almarsson, Ö. & Leiserowitz, L. Quinoline Binding Site on Malaria Pigment Crystal: A Rational Pathway for Antimalaria Drug Design. *Crystal Growth & Design* **2**, 553-562 (2002).

49. Orjih, A., Banyal, H., Chevli, R. & Fitch, C. Hemin Lyses Malaria Parasites. *Science* **214**, 667-669 (1981).

50. Combrinck, J. M. *et al.* Optimization of a Multi-Well Colorimetric Assay to Determine Haem Species in *Plasmodium falciparum* in the Presence of Anti-Malarials. *Malaria Journal* **14**, 253 (2015).

51. Combrinck, J. M. *et al.* Insights into the Role of Heme in the Mechanism of Action of Antimalarials. *ACS Chemical Biology* **8**, 133-137 (2013).

52. Bray, P., Ward, S. & O'Neill, P. Quinolines and Artemisinin: Chemistry, Biology and History. in *Malaria: Drugs, Disease and Post-Genomic Biology* 3-38 (Springer, 2005).

53. Yayon, A., Cabantchik, Z. I. & Ginsburg, H. Susceptibility of Human Malaria Parasites to Chloroquine is pH-Dependent. *Proceedings of the National Academy of Sciences of the United States of America* **82**, 2784-2788 (1985).

54. Ferrari, V. & Cutler, D. J. Simulation of Kinetic Data on the Influx and Efflux of Chloroquine by Erythrocytes Infected with *Plasmodium falciparum*: Evidence for a Drug-Importer in Chloroquine-Sensitive Strains. *Biochemical Pharmacology* **42**, S167-S179 (1991).

55. Egan, T. J. *et al.* Structure–Function Relationships in Aminoquinolines: Effect of Amino and Chloro Groups on Quinoline–Hematin Complex Formation, Inhibition of β-Hematin Formation, and Antiplasmodial Activity. *Journal of Medicinal Chemistry* **43**, 283-291 (2000).

56. Bray, P. G. *et al.* Cellular Uptake of Chloroquine Is Dependent on Binding to Ferriprotoporphyrin IX and Is Independent of NHE Activity in *Plasmodium falciparum. Journal of Cell Biology* **145**, 363-376 (1999).

57. Bray, P. G. *et al.* PfCRT and the Trans-Vacuolar Proton Electrochemical Gradient: Regulating the Access of Chloroquine to Ferriprotoporphyrin IX. *Molecular Microbiology* **62**, 238-251 (2006).

58. Kaschula, C. H. *et al.* Structure–Activity Relationships in 4-Aminoquinoline Antiplasmodials. The Role of the Group at the 7-Position. *Journal of Medicinal Chemistry* **45**, 3531-3539 (2002).

59. Fidock, D. A. *et al.* Mutations in the *P. falciparum* Digestive Vacuole Transmembrane Protein PfCRT and Evidence for Their Role in Chloroquine Resistance. *Molecular Cell* **6**, 861-871 (2000).

60. Martin, R. E. & Kirk, K. The Malaria Parasite's Chloroquine Resistance Transporter is a Member of the Drug/Metabolite Transporter Superfamily. *Molecular Biology and Evolution* **21**, 1938-1949 (2004).

61. Cooper, R. A. *et al.* Alternative Mutations at Position 76 of the Vacuolar Transmembrane Protein PfCRT Are Associated with Chloroquine Resistance and Unique Stereospecific Quinine and Quinidine Responses in *Plasmodium falciparum. Molecular Pharmacology* **61**, 35-42 (2002).

62. Roepe, P. D. PfCRT-Mediated Drug Transport in Malarial Parasites. *Biochemistry* **50**, 163-171 (2011).

63. Martin, R. E. *et al.* Chloroquine Transport via the Malaria Parasite's Chloroquine Resistance Transporter. *Science* **325**, 1680-1682 (2009).

64. Chinappi, M., Via, A., Marcatili, P. & Tramontano, A. On the Mechanism of Chloroquine Resistance in *Plasmodium falciparum. PLOS ONE* **5**, e14064-e14064 (2010).

65. Reed, M. B., Saliba, K. J., Caruana, S. R., Kirk, K. & Cowman, A. F. Pgh1 Modulates Sensitivity and Resistance to Multiple Antimalarials in *Plasmodium falciparum. Nature* **403**, 906-909 (2000).

66. David, H. P. Reversed Chloroquine Molecules as a Strategy to Overcome Resistance in Malaria. *Current Topics in Medicinal Chemistry* **12**, 400-407 (2012).

67. Martiney, J. A., Cerami, A. & Slater, A. F. G. Verapamil Reversal of Chloroquine Resistance in the Malaria Parasite *Plasmodium falciparum* Is Specific for Resistant Parasites and Independent of the Weak Base Effect. *Journal of Biological Chemistry* **270**, 22393-22398 (1995).

68. Bitonti, A. *et al.* Reversal of Chloroquine Resistance in Malaria Parasite *Plasmodium falciparum* by Desipramine. *Science* **242**, 1301-1303 (1988).

69. van Schalkwyk, D. A. & Egan, T. J. Quinoline Resistance Reversing Agents for the Malaria Parasite *Plasmodium falciparum*. *Drug Resistance Updates* **9**, 211-226 (2006).

70. Burgess, S. J. *et al.* A Chloroquine-like Molecule Designed to Reverse Resistance in *Plasmodium falciparum*. *Journal of Medicinal Chemistry* **49**, 5623-5625 (2006).

71. Peyton, D. H. Reversed Chloroquine Molecules as a Strategy to Overcome Resistance in Malaria. *Current Topics in Medicinal Chemistry* **12**, 400-407 (2012).

72. Alibert, S. *et al.* Synthesis and Effects on Chloroquine Susceptibility in *Plasmodium falciparum* of a Series of New Dihydroanthracene Derivatives. *Journal of Medicinal Chemistry* **45**, 3195-3209 (2002).

73. Zishiri, V. K. *et al.* A Series of Structurally Simple Chloroquine Chemosensitizing Dibemethin Derivatives that Inhibit Chloroquine Transport by PfCRT. *European Journal of Medicinal Chemistry* **46**, 1729-1742 (2011).

74. Zishiri, V. K. *et al.* Quinoline Antimalarials Containing a Dibemethin Group Are Active against Chloroquinone-Resistant *Plasmodium falciparum* and Inhibit Chloroquine Transport via the *P. falciparum* Chloroquine-Resistance Transporter (PfCRT). *Journal of Medicinal Chemistry* **54**, 6956-6968 (2011).

75. Joshi, M. C. *et al.* 4-Aminoquinoline Antimalarials Containing a Benzylmethylpyridylmethylamine Group Are Active against Drug-Resistant *Plasmodium falciparum* and Exhibit Oral Activity in Mice. *Journal of Medicinal Chemistry* **60**, 10245-10256 (2017).

76. White, N. J. Cardiotoxicity of Antimalarial Drugs. *The Lancet Infectious Diseases* **7**, 549-558 (2007).

77. Okombo, J. *Physicochemical, Biological And β-Haematin Inhibiting Activity Of Pyridodibemequines, Pyrido[1,2-a]Benzimidazoles And Their Derivatives* PhD thesis, University of Cape Town, (2018).

78. Ding, X. C., Ubben, D. & Wells, T. N. C. A Framework for Assessing the Risk of Resistance for Anti-Malarials in Development. *Malaria Journal* **11**, 292 (2012).

79. Mosmann, T. Rapid Colorimetric Assay for Cellular Growth and Survival: Application to Proliferation and Cytotoxicity Assays. *Journal of Immunological Methods* **65**, 55-63 (1983).

80. Gleeson, M. P. Generation of a Set of Simple, Interpretable ADMET Rules of Thumb. *Journal of Medicinal Chemistry* **51**, 817-834 (2008).

81. Guan, J. *et al.* Design, Synthesis, and Evaluation of New Chemosensitizers in Multi-Drug-Resistant *Plasmodium falciparum*. *Journal of Medicinal Chemistry* **45**, 2741-2748 (2002).

82. Bhattacharjee, A. K., Kyle, D. E., Vennerstrom, J. L. & Milhous, W. K. A 3D QSAR Pharmacophore Model and Quantum Chemical Structure−Activity Analysis of Chloroquine(CQ)-Resistance Reversal. *Journal of Chemical Information and Computer Sciences* **42**, 1212-1220 (2002).

83. Snyder, L. R., Kirkland, J. J. & Glajch, J. L. *Practical HPLC Method Development 2nd ed.*, (John Wiley & Sons, Inc., 1997).

84. Robards, K., Haddad, P. R. & Jackson, P. E. High-Performance Liquid Chromatography - Separations. in *Principles and Practice of Modern Chromatographic Methods 1st ed.* 305-380 (Elsevier Academic Press, 1994).

85. Snyder, L. R., Kirkland, J. J. & Dolan, J. W. *Introduction to Modern Liquid Chromatography 3rd Edition.* (Wiley, 2011).

86. Horvath, C. & Melander, W. Liquid Chromatography with Hydrocarbonaceous Bonded Phases; Theory and Practice of Reversed Phase Chromatography. *Journal of Chromatographic Science* **15**, 393-404 (1977).

87. Snyder, L. R., Dolan, J. W. & Gant, J. R. Gradient Elution in High-Performance Liquid Chromatography: I. Theoretical Basis for Reversed-Phase Systems. *Journal of Chromatography A* **165**, 3-30 (1979).

88. Bidlingmeyer, B. A. Separation of Ionic Compounds by Reversed-Phase Liquid Chromatography An Update of Ion-Pairing Techniques. *Journal of Chromatographic Science* **18**, 525-539 (1980).

89. Ho, C. S. *et al.* Electrospray Ionisation Mass Spectrometry: Principles and Clinical Applications. *The Clinical Biochemist Reviews* **24**, 3-12 (2003).

90. SCIEX. 5500 Series of Instruments System User Guide. (2017).

91. Iribarne, J. V. & Thomson, B. A. On the Evaporation of Small Ions from Charged Droplets. *The Journal of Chemical Physics* **64**, 2287-2294 (1976).

92. Thomson, B. A. & Iribarne, J. V. Field Induced Ion Evaporation from Liquid Surfaces at Atmospheric Pressure. *The Journal of Chemical Physics* **71**, 4451-4463 (1979).

93. Bruins, A. P. Mechanistic Aspects of Electrospray Ionization. *Journal of Chromatography A* **794**, 345-357 (1998).

94. Kebarle, P. & Verkerk, U. H. Electrospray: From Ions in Solution to Ions in the Gas Phase, What We Know Now. *Mass Spectrometry Reviews* **28**, 898-917 (2009).

95. Protein Precipitation: High Throughput Techniques and Strategies for Method Development. in *Progress in Pharmaceutical and Biomedical Analysis* Vol. 5 (ed David A. Wells) Ch. 6, 199-254 (Elsevier, 2003).

96. Li, P. & Bartlett, M. G. A Review of Sample Preparation Methods for Quantitation of Small-Molecule Analytes in Brain Tissue by Liquid Chromatography Tandem Mass Spectrometry (LC-MS/MS). *Analytical Methods* **6**, 6183-6207 (2014).

97. Smith, R. M. Before the Injection—Modern Methods of Sample Preparation for Separation Techniques. *Journal of Chromatography A* **1000**, 3-27 (2003).

98. Bioanalytical Method Validation Guidance for Industry. (U.S. Food and Drug Administration, 2018).

99. Chiu, M. L. *et al.* Matrix Effects—A Challenge toward Automation of Molecular Analysis. *JALA: Journal of the Association for Laboratory Automation* **15**, 233-242 (2010).

100. Bonfiglio, R., King, R. C., Olah, T. V. & Merkle, K. The Effects of Sample Preparation Methods on the Variability of the Electrospray Ionization Response for Model Drug Compounds. *Rapid Communications in Mass Spectrometry* **13**, 1175-1185 (1999).

101. Guideline on Bioanalytical Method Validation. (European Medicines Agency, 2011).

102. Prichard, L. & Barwick, V. *Preparation of Calibration Curves A Guide to Best Practice.* (2003).

103. Van Eeckhaut, A., Lanckmans, K., Sarre, S., Smolders, I. & Michotte, Y. Validation of Bioanalytical LC-MS/MS Assays: Evaluation of Matrix Effects. *Journal of Chromatography B: Analytical Technologies in the Biomedical and Life Sciences* **877**, 2198-2207 (2009).

104. Tan, A., Boudreau, N. & Lévesque, A. Internal Standards for Quantitative LC-MS Bioanalysis. in *LC-MS in Drug Bioanalysis* (eds Q. Alan Xu & Timothy L. Madden) Ch. 1, 1-32 (Springer US, 2012).

105. Hughes, N. C., Wong, E. Y., Fan, J. & Bajaj, N. Determination of Carryover and Contamination for Mass Spectrometry-Based Chromatographic Assays. *AAPS Journal* **9**, E353-E360 (2007).

106. King, R., Bonfiglio, R., Fernandez-Metzler, C., Miller-Stein, C. & Olah, T. Mechanistic Investigation of Ionization Suppression in Electrospray Ionization. *Journal of the American Society for Mass Spectrometry* **11**, 942-950 (2000).

107. Trufelli, H., Palma, P., Famiglini, G. & Cappiello, A. An Overview of Matrix Effects in Liquid Chromatography-Mass Spectrometry. *Mass Spectrometry Reviews* **30**, 491-509 (2011).

108. Gosetti, F., Mazzucco, E., Zampieri, D. & Gennaro, M. C. Signal Suppression/Enhancement in High-Performance Liquid Chromatography Tandem Mass Spectrometry. *Journal of Chromatography A* **1217**, 3929-3937 (2010).

109. Matuszewski, B. K., Constanzer, M. L. & Chavez-Eng, C. M. Strategies for the Assessment of Matrix Effect in Quantitative Bioanalytical Methods Based on HPLC-MS/MS. *Analytical Chemistry* **75**, 3019-3030 (2003).

110. Briscoe, C. J. & Hage, D. S. Factors Affecting the Stability of Drugs and Drug Metabolites in Biological Matrices. *Bioanalysis* **1**, 205-220 (2009).

111. Reed, G. A. Stability of Drugs, Drug Candidates, and Metabolites in Blood and Plasma. *Current Protocols in Pharmacology* **75**, 7.6.1-7.6.12 (2016).

112. Shabihkhani, M. *et al.* The Procurement, Storage, and Quality Assurance of Frozen Blood and Tissue Biospecimens in Pathology, Biorepository, and Biobank Settings. *Clinical Biochemistry* **47**, 258-266 (2014).

113. Shimizu, Y. & Ichihara, K. Elucidation of Stability Profiles of Common Chemistry Analytes in Serum Stored at Six Graded Temperatures. *Clinical Chemisty and Laboratory Medicine* **57**, 1388-1396 (2019).

114. van de Merbel, N. *et al.* Stability: Recommendation for Best Practices and Harmonization from the Global Bioanalysis Consortium Harmonization Team. *The AAPS Journal* **16**, 392-399 (2014).

115. Peng, L. & Farkas, T. Analysis of Basic Compounds by Reversed-Phase Liquid Chromatography–Electrospray Mass Spectrometry in High-pH Mobile Phases. *Journal of Chromatography A* **1179**, 131-144 (2008).

116. Zhou, S., Prebyl, B. S. & Cook, K. D. Profiling pH Changes in the Electrospray Plume. *Analytical Chemistry* **74**, 4885-4888 (2002).

117. Phenomenex. Gemini pH Flexibility. (2015).

118. Katzung, B. G., Masters, S. B. & Trevor, A. J. Pharmacokinetics and Pharmacodynamics: Rational Dosing & the Time Course of Drug Action. in *Basic & Clinical Pharmacology 12th ed.* 37–49 (McGraw-Hill Medical, 2012).

119. Wang, J., Urban, L. & Bojanic, D. Maximising Use of *in vitro* ADMET Tools to Predict *in vivo* Bioavailability and Safety. *Expert Opinion on Drug Metabolism & Toxicology* **3**, 641-665 (2007).

120. Li, C. *et al.* A Modern in vivo Pharmacokinetic Paradigm: Combining Snapshot, Rapid and Full PK Approaches to Optimize and Expedite Early Drug Discovery. *Drug Discovey Today* **18**, 71-78 (2013).

121. Kwon, Y. Pharmacokinetic Study Design and Data Interpretation. In *Handbook of Essential Pharmacokinetics, Pharmacodynamics and Drug Metabolism for Industrial Scientists 1st ed.* 3-28 (Springer, 2002).

122. Evans, D. F. *et al.* Measurement of Gastrointestinal pH Profiles in Normal Ambulant Human Subjects. *Gut* **29**, 1035-1041 (1988).

123. Amidon, G. L., Lennernas, H., Shah, V. P. & Crison, J. R. Theoretical Basis for a Biopharmaceutic Drug Classification: The Correlation of in Vitro Drug Product Dissolution and in Vivo Bioavailability. *Pharmaceutical Research* **12**, 413-420 (1995).

124. Hansen, N. T., Kouskoumvekaki, I., Jørgensen, F. S., Brunak, S. & Jónsdóttir, S. Ó. Prediction of pH-Dependent Aqueous Solubility of Druglike Molecules. *Journal of Chemical Information and Modeling* **46**, 2601–2609 (2006).

125. Lipinski, C. A., Lombardo, F., Dominy, B. W. & Feeney, P. J. Experimental and Computational Approaches to Estimate Solubility and Permeability in Drug Discovery and Development Settings. *Advanced Drug Delivery Reviews* **23**, 3–25 (1997).

126. Li, S. *et al.* Enhanced Bioavailability of a Poorly Water-Soluble Weakly Basic Compound Using a Combination Approach of Solubilization Agents and Precipitation Inhibitors: A Case Study. *Molecular Pharmaceutics* **9**, 1100-1108 (2012).

127. Cairns, D. Physicochemical Properties of Drugs. in *Essentials of Pharmaceutical Chemistry 4th ed.* 57–79 (Pharmaceutical Press, 2012).

128. Katzung, B. G., Masters, S. B. & Trevor, A. J. Drug Biotransformation. in *Basic & Clinical Pharmacology 12th ed.* 53–68 (McGraw-Hill Medical, 2012).

129. Brunton, L. L., Lazo, J. S. & Parker, K. L. Drug Metabolism. in *Goodman & Gilman's The Pharmacological Basis of Therapeutics 11th ed.* 71-91 (McGraw Hill, 2006).

130. Kerns, E. H. & Di, L. Plasma Protein Binding. in *Drug-like Properties: Concepts, Structure Design and Methods: from ADME to Toxicity Optimization 1st Ed.* 187–196 (Academic Press, 2008).

131. Smith, D. A., Di, L. & Kerns, E. H. The Effect of Plasma Protein Binding on *In Vivo* Efficacy: Misconceptions in Drug Discovery. *Nature Reviews Drug Discovery* **9**, 929–939 (2010).

132. Kansy, M., Senner, F. & Gubernator, K. Physicochemical High Throughput Screening: Parallel Artificial Membrane Permeation Assay in the Description of Passive Absorption Processes. *Journal of Medicinal Chemistry* **41**, 1007-1010 (1998).

133. Kerns, E. H. & Di, L. Permeability Methods. in *Drug-like Properties: Concepts, Structure Design and Methods: from ADME to Toxicity Optimization 1st Ed.* 287-298 (Academic Press, 2008).

134. Yan, Z. & Caldwell, G. W. Metabolism Profiling, and Cytochrome P450 Inhibition & Induction in Drug Discovery. *Current Topics in Medicinal Chemistry* **1**, 403–425 (2001).

135. Kerns, E. H. & Di, L. Metabolic Stability Methods. in *Drug-like Properties: Concepts, Structure Design and Methods: from ADME to Toxicity Optimization 1st Ed.* 329-347 (Academic Press, 2008).

136. Gabrielsson, J. & Weiner, D. Non-compartmental Analysis. *Methods in Molecular Biology* **929**, 377–389 (2012).

137. Brock-Utne, J. G. & Kingston, H. G. G. Basic Pharmacokinetics. *South African Medical Journal* **58**, 361–365 (1980).

138. Jambhekar, S. S. & Breen, P. J. Extravascular Routes of Drug Administration. In *Basic Pharmacokinetics 2nd ed.* 105–126 (Pharmaceutical Press, 2012).

139. Urso, R., Blardi, P. & Giorgi, G. A Short Introduction to Pharmacokinetics. *European Review for Medical and Pharmacological Sciences* **6**, 33-44 (2002).

140. Fan, J.-H. & Lannoy, I. A. M. D. Pharmacokinetics. *Biochemical Pharmacology* **87**, 93–120 (2014).

141. Benet, L. Z. & Zia-Amirhosseini, P. Basic Principles of Pharmacokinetics. *Toxicologic Pathology* **23**, 115–123 (1995).

142. Bakshi, R. P., Nenortas, E., Tripathi, A. K., Sullivan, D. J. & Shapiro, T. A. Model System to Define Pharmacokinetic Requirements for Antimalarial Drug Efficacy. *Science Translational Medicine* **5**, 205ra135 (2013).

143. Tuntland, T. *et al.* Implementation of Pharmacokinetic and Pharmacodynamic Strategies in Early Research Phases of Drug Discovery and Development at Novartis Institute of Biomedical Research. *Frontiers in Pharmacology* **5**, 1-16 (2014).

144. Lakshminarayana, S. B. *et al.* Pharmacokinetic-Pharmacodynamic Analysis of Spiroindolone Analogs and KAE609 in a Murine Malaria Model. *Antimicrobial Agents and Chemotherapy* **59**, 1200-1210 (2015).

145. Zhang, Y., Huo, M., Zhou, J. & Xie, S. PKSolver: An Add-In Program for Pharmacokinetic and Pharmacodynamic Data Analysis in Microsoft Excel. *Computer Methods and Programs in Biomedicine* **99**, 306–314 (2010).

146. Bergqvist, Y. & Domeij-Nyberg, B. Distribution of Chloroquine and its Metabolite Desethyl-Chloroquine in Human Blood Cells and its Implication for the Quantitative Determination of these Compounds in Serum and Plasma. *Journal of Chromatography* **272**, 137-148 (1983).

147. Baggot, J. D. Pharmacokinetic-Pharmacodynamic Relationship. *Annales de Recherches Veterinaires.* **21** 29s-40s (1990).

148. Rohatagi, S., Martin, N. E. & Barrett, J. S. Pharmacokinetic/Pharmacodynamic Modeling in Drug Development. In *Applications of Pharmacokinetic Principles in Drug Development* (ed Rajesh Krishna) 333-372 (Springer US, 2004).

149. White, N. J. Pharmacokinetic and Pharmacodynamic Considerations in Antimalarial Dose Optimization. *Antimicrobial Agents and Chemotherapy* **57**, 5792–5807 (2013).

150. White, N. J. *et al.* Malaria. *The Lancet* **383**, 723-735 (2014).

151. Lotharius, J. *et al.* Repositioning: the Fast Track to New Anti-Malarial Medicines? *Malaria Journal* **13**, 143 (2014).

152. Moreno, A., Pérignon, J. L., Morosan, S., Mazier, D. & Benito, A. *Plasmodium falciparum*-Infected Mice: More than a Tour de Force. *Trends in Parasitology* **23**, 254-259 (2007).

153. Moreno-Sabater, A., Pérignon, J. L., Mazier, D., Lavazec, C. & Soulard, V. Humanized Mouse Models Infected with Human *Plasmodium* Species for Antimalarial Drug Discovery. *Expert Opinion on Drug Discovery* **13**, 131-140 (2018).

154. Ito, M. *et al.* NOD/SCID/γnullc Mouse: An Excellent Recipient Mouse Model for Engraftment of Human Cells. *Blood* **100**, 3175-3182 (2002).

155. Arnold, L. *et al.* Further Improvements of the *P. falciparum* Humanized Mouse Model. *PLOS ONE* **6**, e18045 (2011).

156. Brehm, M. A., Wiles, M. V., Greiner, D. L. & Shultz, L. D. Generation of Improved Humanized Mouse Models for Human Infectious Diseases. *Journal of Immunological Methods* **410**, 3-17 (2014).

157. Jiménez-Díaz, M. B. *et al.* Improved Murine Model of Malaria Using *Plasmodium falciparum* Competent Strains and Non-Myelodepleted NOD-scid IL2Rγnull Mice Engrafted with Human Erythrocytes. *Antimicrobial Agents and Chemotherapy* **53**, 4533-4536 (2009).

158. Angulo-Barturen, I. *et al.* A Murine Model of *P. falciparum*-Malaria by *In Vivo* Selection of Competent Strains in Non-Myelodepleted Mice Engrafted with Human Erythrocytes. *PLOS ONE* **3**, e2252 (2008).

159. Introduction to Flow Cytometry: A Learning Guide. (Becton, Dickinson and Company, USA, 2002).

160. Givan, A. L. *Flow Cytometry: First Principles 2nd ed.*, (John Wiley & Sons, 2013).

161. Jiménez-Díaz, M. B. *et al.* Quantitative Measurement of *Plasmodium*-Infected Erythrocytes in Murine Models of Malaria by Flow Cytometry using Bidimensional Assessment of SYTO-16 Fluorescence. *Cytometry Part A* **75A**, 225-235 (2009).

162. Kina, T. *et al.* The Monoclonal Antibody TER-119 Recognizes a Molecule Associated with Glycophorin A and Specifically Marks the Late Stages of Murine Erythroid Lineage. *British Journal of Haematology* **109**, 280-287 (2000).

163. Arnot, D. E. & Gull, K. The *Plasmodium* Cell-Cycle: Facts and Questions. *Annals of Tropical Medicine and Parasitology* **92**, 361-365 (1998).

164. Stanojcic, S., Kuk, N., Ullah, I., Sterkers, Y. & Merrick, C. J. Single-Molecule Analysis Reveals that DNA Replication Dynamics Vary Across the Course of Schizogony in the Malaria Parasite *Plasmodium falciparum*. *Scientific Reports* **7**, 4003 (2017).

165. Chevalley, S., Coste, A., Lopez, A., Pipy, B. & Valentin, A. Flow Cytometry for the Evaluation of Anti-Plasmodial Activity of Drugs on *Plasmodium falciparum* Gametocytes. *Malaria Journal* **9**, 49 (2010).

166. Grimberg, B. T., Erickson, J. J., Sramkoski, R. M., Jacobberger, J. W. & Zimmerman, P. A. Monitoring *Plasmodium falciparum* Growth and Development by UV Flow Cytometry using an Optimized Hoechst-Thiazole Orange Staining Strategy. *Cytometry Part A* **73A**, 546-554 (2008).

167. Peters, W., Portus, J. H. & Robinson, B. L. The Chemotherapy of Rodent Malaria, XXII. *Annals of Tropical Medicine & Parasitology* **69**, 155-171 (1975).

168. Foley, M. & Tilley, L. Quinoline Antimalarials: Mechanisms of Action and Resistance and Prospects for New Agents. *Pharmacology & Therapeutics* **79**, 55-87 (1998).

169. Gibhard, L. *et al.* Investigating Sulfoxide-to-Sulfone Conversion as a Prodrug Strategy for a Phosphatidylinositol 4-Kinase Inhibitor in a Humanized Mouse Model of Malaria. *Antimicrobial Agents and Chemotherapy* **62**, e00261-00218 (2018).

170. MacDougall, J. Analysis of Dose-Response Studies-Emax Model. in *Dose Finding in Drug Development Ed. 1* (ed Naitee Ting) Ch. 9, 137-135 (Springer, 2006).

171. Le Manach, C. *et al.* Medicinal Chemistry Optimization of Antiplasmodial Imidazopyridazine Hits from High Throughput Screening of a SoftFocus Kinase Library: Part 1. *Journal of Medicinal Chemistry* **57**, 2789-2798 (2014).

172. White, N. Antimalarial Drug Resistance and Combination Chemotherapy. *Philosophical Transactions of the Royal Society of London Series B* **354**, 739-749 (1999).

173. Hastings, I. M. A Model for the Origins and Spread of Drug-Resistant Malaria. *Parasitology* **115** 133-142 (1997).

174. Peters, W. The Prevention of Antimalarial Drug Resistance. *Pharmacology & Therapeutics* **47**, 499-508 (1990).

175. Matthews, H., Deakin, J., Rajab, M., Idris-Usman, M. & Nirmalan, N. J. Investigating Antimalarial Drug Interactions of Emetine Dihydrochloride Hydrate using CalcuSyn-Based Interactivity Calculations. *PLOS ONE* **12**, 1-19 (2017).

176. Chou, T.-C. Theoretical Basis, Experimental Design, and Computerized Simulation of Synergism and Antagonism in Drug Combination Studies. *Pharmacological Reviews* **58**, 621-681 (2006).

177. Bell, A. Antimalarial Drug Synergism and Antagonism: Mechanistic and Clinical Significance. *FEMS Microbiology Letters* **253**, 171-184 (2005).

178. Gorka, A. P., Jacobs, L. M. & Roepe, P. D. Cytostatic Versus Cytocidal Profiling of Quinoline Drug Combinations Via Modified Fixed-Ratio Isobologram Analysis. *Malaria Journal* **12**, 332 (2013).

179. Breitinger, H.-G. Drug Synergy – Mechanisms and Methods of Analysis. in *Toxicity and Drug Testing 1st ed.* (ed William Acree) 143-166 (IntechOpen, 2012).

180. Watkins, W. M. & Mosobo, M. Treatment of *Plasmodium falciparum* Malaria with Pyrimethamine-Sulfadoxine: Selective Pressure for Resistance is a Function of Long Elimination Half-Life. *Transactions of The Royal Society of Tropical Medicine and Hygiene* **87**, 75-78 (1993).

181. Combrinck, J. *The Role Of Haem In The Mechanism Of Action Of Antimalarials In Plasmodium falciparum* PhD thesis, University of Cape Town, (2016).

182. Dhingra, S. K. *et al.* A Variant PfCRT Isoform Can Contribute to *Plasmodium falciparum* Resistance to the First-Line Partner Drug Piperaquine. *mBio* **8**, 1-19 (2017).

183. Moore, L. R. *et al.* Hemoglobin Degradation in Malaria-Infected Erythrocytes Determined from Live Cell Magnetophoresis. *The FASEB Journal* **20**, 747-749 (2006).

184. Terkuile, F., White, N. J., Holloway, P., Pasvol, G. & Krishna, S. *Plasmodium falciparum: In Vitro* Studies of the Pharmacodynamic Properties of Drugs Used for the Treatment of Severe Malaria. *Experimental Parasitology* **76**, 85-95 (1993).

185. Sanchez, C. P., Rotmann, A., Stein, W. D. & Lanzer, M. Polymorphisms within PfMDR1 Alter the Substrate Specificity for Anti-Malarial Drugs in *Plasmodium falciparum*. *Molecular Microbiology* **70**, 786-798 (2008).

186. Haynes, R. & Vonwiller, S. The Behavior of Qinghaosu (Artemisinin) in the Presence of Heme Iron(II) and (III). *Tetrahedron Letters* **37**, 253-256 (1996).

187. Wu, W.-M. *et al.* Unified Mechanistic Framework for the Fe(II)-Induced Cleavage of Qinghaosu and Derivatives/Analogues. The First Spin-Trapping Evidence for the Previously Postulated Secondary C-4 Radical. *Journal of the American Chemical Society* **120**, 3316-3325 (1998).

188. Bridgford, J. L. *et al.* Artemisinin Kills Malaria Parasites by Damaging Proteins and Inhibiting the Proteasome. *Nature Communications* **9**, 1-11 (2018).

189. Olliaro, P. L., Haynes, R. K., Meunier, B. & Yuthavong, Y. Possible Modes of Action of the Artemisinin-Type Compounds. *Trends in Parasitology* **17**, 122-126 (2001).

190. Mbengue, A. *et al.* A Molecular Mechanism of Artemisinin Resistance in *Plasmodium falciparum* Malaria. *Nature* **520**, 683-687 (2015).

191. Wilson, D. W., Langer, C., Goodman, C. D., McFadden, G. I. & Beeson, J. G. Defining the Timing of Action of Antimalarial Drugs against *Plasmodium falciparum*. *Antimicrobial Agents and Chemotherapy* **57**, 1455-1467 (2013).

192. Ariey, F. *et al.* A Molecular Marker of Artemisinin-Resistant *Plasmodium falciparum* Malaria. *Nature* **505**, 50-55 (2014).

193. Sanz, L. M. *et al. P. falciparum In Vitro* Killing Rates Allow to Discriminate between Different Antimalarial Mode-of-Action. *PLOS ONE* **7**, 1-11 (2012).

194. Wong, W. *et al.* Mefloquine Targets The *Plasmodium falciparum* 80S Ribosome to Inhibit Protein Synthesis. *Nature Microbiology* **2**, 1-9 (2017).

195. Price, R. N. *et al.* Mefloquine Resistance in *Plasmodium falciparum* and Increased pfmdr1 Gene Copy Number. *Lancet* **364**, 438-447 (2004).

196. Sanchez, C. P., Dave, A., Stein, W. D. & Lanzer, M. Transporters as Mediators of Drug Resistance in *Plasmodium falciparum*. *International Journal for Parasitology* **40**, 1109-1118 (2010).

197. Sisowath, C. *et al. In Vivo* Selection of *Plasmodium falciparum* Parasites Carrying the Chloroquine-Susceptible pfcrt K76 Allele after Treatment with Artemether-Lumefantrine in Africa. *The Journal of Infectious Diseases* **199**, 750-757 (2009).

198. Mungthin, M. *et al.* Association Between the pfmdr1 Gene and In Vitro Artemether and Lumefantrine Sensitivity in Thai Isolates of *Plasmodium falciparum*. *The American Society of Tropical Medicine and Hygiene* **83**, 1005-1009 (2010).

199. Sidhu, A. B. S. *et al.* Decreasing pfmdr1 Copy Number in *Plasmodium falciparum* Malaria Heightens Susceptibility to Mefloquine, Lumefantrine, Halofantrine, Quinine, and Artemisinin. *The Journal of Infectious Diseases* **194**, 528-535 (2006).

200. Färber, P. M., Arscott, L. D., Williams, C. H., Becker, K. & Schirmer, R. H. Recombinant *Plasmodium falciparum* Glutathione Reductase is Inhibited by the Antimalarial Dye Methylene Blue. *FEBS Letters* **422**, 311-314 (1998).

201. Atamna, H. *et al.* Mode of Antimalarial Effect of Methylene Blue and some of its Analogues on *Plasmodium falciparum* in Culture and their Inhibition of *P. vinckei petteri* and *P. yoelii nigeriensis in vivo*. *Biochemical Pharmacology* **51**, 693-700 (1996).

202. Akoachere, M. *et al.* In Vitro Assessment of Methylene Blue on Chloroquine-Sensitive and -Resistant *Plasmodium falciparum* Strains Reveals Synergistic Action with Artemisinins. *Antimicrobial Agents and Chemotherapy* **49**, 4592-4597 (2005).

203. Garavito, G. *et al.* Blood Schizontocidal Activity of Methylene Blue in Combination with Antimalarials against *Plasmodium falciparum. Parasite* **14**, 135-140 (2007).

204. Thurston, J. P. The Chemotherapy of *Plasmodium berghei.* I. Resistance to Drugs. *Parasitology* **43**, 246-252 (1953).

205. Lu, G. *et al.* Efficacy and Safety of Methylene Blue in the Treatment of Malaria: a Systematic Review. *BMC Medicine* **16**, 1-16 (2018).

206. Fry, M. & Pudney, M. Site of Action of the Antimalarial Hydroxynaphthoquinone, 2-[trans-4-(4'-Chlorophenyl) Cyclohexyl]-3- Hydroxy-1,4-Naphthoquinone (566C80). *Biochemical Pharmacology* **43**, 1545-1553 (1992).

207. Srivastava, I. K., Rottenberg, H. & Vaidya, A. B. Atovaquone, a Broad Spectrum Antiparasitic Drug, Collapses Mitochondrial Membrane Potential in a Malarial Parasite. *Journal of Biological Chemistry* **272**, 3961-3966 (1997).

208. Painter, H. J., Morrisey, J. M., Mather, M. W. & Vaidya, A. B. Specific Role of Mitochondrial Electron Transport in Blood-Stage *Plasmodium falciparum. Nature* **446**, 88-91 (2007).

209. Srivastava, I. K., Morrisey, J. M., Darrouzet, E., Daldal, F. & Vaidya, A. B. Resistance Mutations Reveal The Atovaquone-Binding Domain of Cytochrome B in Malaria Parasites. *Molecular Microbiology* **33**, 704-711 (1999).

210. Elion, G. B., Singer, S. & Hitchings, G. H. Antagonists of Nucleic Acid Derivatives: Synergism in Combinations of Biochemically Related Antimetabolites. *Journal of Biological Chemistry* **208**, 477-488 (1953).

211. Hsieh, M. H., Yu, C. M., Yu, V. L. & Chow, J. W. Synergy Assessed by Checkerboard a Critical Analysis. *Diagnostic Microbiology and Infectious Disease* **16**, 343-349 (1993).

212. Chou, T.-C. & Talalay, P. Quantitative Analysis of Dose-Effect Relationships: The Combined Effects of Multiple Drugs or Enzyme Inhibitors. *Advances in enzyme regulation* **22**, 27-55 (1984).

213. Loewe, S. The Problem of Synergism and Antagonism of Combined Drugs. *Arzneimittelforschung [Drug Research]* **3**, 285-290 (1953).

214. Greco, W. R., Bravo, G. & Parsons, J. C. The Search for Synergy: A Critical Review from a Response Surface Perspective. *Pharmacological Reviews* **47**, 331-385 (1995).

215. Fivelman, Q. L., Adagu, I. S. & Warhurst, D. C. Modified Fixed-Ratio Isobologram Method for Studying *In Vitro* Interactions between Atovaquone and Proguanil or Dihydroartemisinin against Drug-Resistant Strains of *Plasmodium falciparum*. *Antimicrobial Agents and Chemotherapy* **48**, 4097-4102 (2004).

216. Huang, R.-y. *et al.* Isobologram Analysis: A Comprehensive Review of Methodology and Current Research. *Frontiers in Pharmacology* **10**, 1-12 (2019).

217. Berenbaum, M. C. A Method for Testing for Synergy with Any Number of Agents. *The Journal of Infectious Diseases* **137**, 122-130 (1978).

218. Abiodun, O. O., Brun, R. & Wittlin, S. *In Vitro* Interaction of Artemisinin Derivatives or the Fully Synthetic Peroxidic Anti-Malarial OZ277 with Thapsigargin in *Plasmodium falciparum* Strains. *Malaria Journal* **12**, 43-46 (2013).

219. Snyder, C., Chollet, J., Santo-Tomas, J., Scheurer, C. & Wittlin, S. *In Vitro* and *In Vivo* Interaction of Synthetic Peroxide RBx11160 (OZ277) with Piperaquine in *Plasmodium* Models. *Experimental Parasitology* **115**, 296-300 (2007).

220. Ibraheem, Z. O., Abd Majid, R., Noor, S. M., Sedik, H. M. & Basir, R. Role of Different Pfcrt and Pfmdr-1 Mutations in Conferring Resistance to Antimalaria Drugs in *Plasmodium falciparum*. *Malaria Research and Treatment* **2014**, 1-17 (2014).

221. Chugh, M. *et al.* Identification and Deconvolution of Cross-Resistance Signals from Antimalarial Compounds Using Multidrug-Resistant *Plasmodium falciparum* Strains. *Antimicrobial Agents and Chemotherapy* **59**, 1110-1118 (2015).

222. Trager, W. & Jensen, J. B. Human Malaria Parasites in Continuous Culture. *Science* **193**, 673-675 (1976).

223. Lambros, C. & Vanderberg, J. P. Synchronization of *Plasmodium falciparum* Erythrocytic Stages in Culture. *The Journal of Parasitology* **65**, 418-420 (1979).

224. Makler, M. T. & Hinrichs, D. J. Measurement of the Lactate Dehydrogenase Activity of *Plasmodium falciparum* as an Assessment of Parasitemia. *The American Journal of Tropical Medicine and Hygiene* **48**, 205-210 (1993).

225. Klonis, N. *et al.* Artemisinin activity against *Plasmodium falciparum* requires hemoglobin uptake and digestion. *Proceedings of the National Academy of Sciences* **108**, 11405-11410 (2011).

226. Wang, J. *et al.* Haem-Activated Promiscuous Targeting of Artemisinin in *Plasmodium falciparum*. *Nature Communications* **6**, 1-11 (2015).

227. Fivelman, Q. L., Adagu, I. S. & Warhurst, D. C. Effects of Piperaquine, Chloroquine, and Amodiaquine on Drug Uptake and of These in Combination with Dihydroartemisinin against Drug-Sensitive and -Resistant *Plasmodium falciparum* Strains. *Antimicrobial Agents and Chemotherapy* **51**, 2265-2267 (2007).

228. Fitch, C. D., Chan, R. L. & Chevli, R. Chloroquine Resistance in Malaria: Accessibility of Drug Receptors to Mefloquine. *Antimicrobial Agents Chemotherapy* **15**, 258-262 (1979).

229. Geary, T. G., Bonanni, L. C., B.Jensen, J. & Ginsburg, H. Effects of Combinations of Quinoline-Containing Antimalarials on *Plasmodium falciparum* in Culture. *Annals of Tropical Medicine & Parasitology* **80**, 285-291 (1986).

230. Famin, O. & Ginsburg, H. Differential Effects of 4-Aminoquinoline-Containing Antimalarial Drugs on Hemoglobin Digestion in *Plasmodium falciparum*-Infected Erythrocytes. *Biochemical Pharmacology* **63**, 393-398 (2002).

231. Vanderkooi, G., Prapunwattana, P. & Yuthavong, Y. Evidence for Electrogenic Accumulation of Mefloquine by Malarial Parasites. *Biochemical Pharmacology* **37**, 3623-3631 (1988).

232. Kerns, E. H., Di, L. & Carter, G. T. *In Vitro* Solubility Assays in Drug Discovery. *Current Drug Metabolism* **9**, 879-885 (2008).

233. Buscher, B. *et al.* Bioanalysis for Plasma Protein Binding Studies in Drug Discovery and Drug Development: Views and Recommendations of the European Bioanalysis Forum. *Bioanalysis* **6**, 673-682 (2014).

234. Wein, S. *et al.* New Insight into the Mechanism of Accumulation and Intraerythrocytic Compartmentation of Albitiazolium, a New Type of Antimalarial. *Antimicrobial Agents and Chemotherapy* **58**, 5519-5527 (2014).

235. Hawley, S. R. *et al.* Relationship between Antimalarial Drug Activity, Accumulation, and Inhibition of Heme Polymerization in *Plasmodium falciparum in vitro*. *Antimicrobial Agents and Chemotherapy* **42**, 682-686 (1998).

236. Ouédraogo, A. L. *et al.* A Protocol for Membrane Feeding Assays to Determine the Infectiousness of *P. falciparum* Naturally Infected Individuals to *Anopheles gambiae*. *Malaria World Journal* **4**, 1-4 (2013).

237. Derbyshire, E. R., Prudêncio, M., Mota, M. M. & Clardy, J. Liver-Stage Malaria Parasites Vulnerable to Diverse Chemical Scaffolds. *Proceedings of the National Academy of Sciences* **109**, 8511-8516 (2012).

238. Daher, W. *et al.* Assessment of *Plasmodium falciparum* Resistance to Ferroquine (SSR97193) in Field Isolates and in W2 Strain Under Pressure. *Malaria Journal* **5**, 11 (2006).

239. Blasco, B., Leroy, D. & Fidock, D. A. Antimalarial Drug Resistance: Linking *Plasmodium falciparum* Parasite Biology to the Clinic. *Nature Medicine* **23**, 917-928 (2017).

240. Ammerman, N. C., Beier-Sexton, M. & Azad, A. F. Growth and Maintenance of Vero Cell Lines. *Current Protocols in Microbiology* **11**, A.4E.1-A.4E.7 (2008).

241. Ames, B. N., Durston, W. E., Yamasaki, E. & Lee, F. D. Carcinogens are Mutagens: A Simple Test System Combining Liver Homogenates for Activation and Bacteria for Detection. *Proceedings of the National Academy of Sciences* **70**, 2281-2285 (1973).

242. Danker, T. & Möller, C. Early Identification of hERG Liability in Drug Discovery Programs by Automated Patch Clamp. *Frontiers in Pharmacology* **5** (2014).

243. Li, G., Huang, K., Nikolic, D. & van Breemen, R. B. High-Throughput Cytochrome P450 Cocktail Inhibition Assay for Assessing Drug-Drug and Drug-Botanical Interactions. *Drug Metabolism and Disposition* **43**, 1670-1678 (2015).

244. Beutler, E. & Duparc, S. Glucose-6-Phosphate Dehydrogenase Deficiency and Antimalarial Drug Development. *The American Journal of Tropical Medicine and Hygiene* **77**, 779-789 (2007).

www.ingramcontent.com/pod-product-compliance
Lightning Source LLC
LaVergne TN
LVHW091154150826
845672LV00005B/1145
* 9 7 8 3 3 8 4 2 7 0 6 5 8 *

Praise for *The Space Between Summits*

"Get ready for a journey of keen awareness of the opposites in life that often reside in the same space: being fragile yet strong, fearful but unafraid, broken yet healing, lost while discovering self. Filled with stories of adventure that helped one woman navigate heartbreaking loss, *The Space Between Summits* teaches us how fragile life is yet is a shining example of how fearlessly living life on the edge connects us with the world and our inner selves, and ultimately, leads to healing."

—Marshall Ulrich, adventurer and bestselling author of *Running on Empty* and *Both Feet on the Ground*

"Adventure racing and climbing Everest gave me a real appreciation for Dianette's mental tenacity and physical endurance. *The Space Between Summits* is her personal spiritual journey that she willingly shares with us. Climbing the highest mountain in Antarctica with Johnny Strange when he was twelve and bumping into him at the North Pole years later gives me a unique perspective on him. We spoke of passion and risk, and how he wanted to live his life as fully as possible. With their shared 'Life Wish' ever present, *The Space Between Summits* is truly a love story."

—Vern Tejas, mountain guide

"No one I know has the courage to explore the world and the limits of herself. A must read!"

—Gerald W. Abrams, executive producer

"I really loved the book—so impressive! I am humbled. *The Space Between Summits* beautifully illustrates the resilience with which Dianette approached each challenge in her life."

—Mary Gadams, founder of RacingThePlanet

"What a ride! In *The Space Between Summits*, Dianette takes you to the top of the world and the depths of the soul as she reminds us every day is training day for the challenges, sorrow, boundless joy, and intense beauty that true adventure and the search for meaning and purpose bring. Biting wit and gallows humor combined with compassion and heart—Dianette and her story will help get you up and down any mountain."

—Kelly Chapman Meyer, founder of OneSun Farms

"Dianette's life is rife with summits and valleys, and completing this book is a testament to living her truth—living authentically and with joy in *The Space Between Summits.*"

**—Laureen Nolan Sills, founder of
Malibu Special Education Foundation**

"Dianette is a force of nature. Whether she's climbing the highest mountains or tackling the massive challenge of writing a book, she tells her story of triumph and tragedy with style and courage. What a fantastic achievement."

—John Watkin, Emmy-winning producer/director